THE ROSACEA HANDBOOK

A SELF-HELP GUIDE

BY

ANN-MARIE LINDSTROM

United Research Publishers

Published by United Research Publishers
Printed and bound in the United States of America
ISBN 1-887053-14-X
Library of Congress Control Number 00-131566
Copyright © 2000 by United Research Publishers

The information in this book is not intended to replace the advice of your physician. You should
consult your doctor regarding any medical condition
which concerns you. The material presented in this
book is intended to inform and educate the reader
with a view to making some intelligent choices in
pursuing the goal of living your life in a healthy, vigorous manner.

Order additional copies from:

United Research Publishers
P.O. Box 232344
Encinitas, CA 92023-2344

or:

www.unitedresearchpubs.com

Full 90-day money back guarantee if not satisfied.

My most sincere thanks to the National Rosacea Society for the use of their statistics and photos.

TABLE OF
CONTENTS

INTRODUCTION

One Thanksgiving, we went to Arizona for a family dinner. The sun was bright, but the wind was chilly on the high desert. On Sunday afternoon, as we said our good-byes and headed for the freeways and airports, someone tried to wipe some lipstick off my cheek.

I flipped down the visor mirror once we were on the road. Both cheeks were rosy. Not pink rosy—more like American Beauty rosy. That deep red is lovely on long stems, in a vase. It wasn't so attractive on my face. I figured I had a winter sun/wind burn. Wondered if I could tell people back home I'd been skiing in Aspen.

I was busy with work and Christmas preparations for the next couple weeks, and didn't pay much attention to my face. Some days the color seemed to be fading. Sunburn in December isn't common in Southern California, but I figured it wasn't impossible.

Then I noticed some small white bumps. Not quite pimples. Since I had been battling a couple patches of eczema on my leg for months, I panicked. I assumed it had spread to my face. While I could cope (not graciously) with weeping flesh under my pants' legs, I wasn't ready to go about my daily life with a bag over my head. I raced to the dermatologist.

He told me I only had rosacea and gave me a small tube of cream. I vaguely remembered having heard of something called rosacea. The cream worked. The white bumps disappeared, and my skin returned to its natural color. I didn't give the whole thing much thought.

One night a few months later, I was researching something else on the Internet and entered rosacea into the search engine. After two hours of reading, I wasn't so complacent about rosacea. It was a shock to find out I was a victim of an incurable, progressive disease. That phrase ran through my head for days. I'd never had an incurable, progressive disease before.

Soon, other thoughts intruded—like making a living and dealing with daily life. My skin returned to normal, without cream. The tube of cream disappeared into the black hole under the bathroom sink.

When my publisher mentioned he was considering putting out a book about rosacea, I jumped up and down, waving my arm—I'll do it. I'll do it.

The research was fascinating. I got to rummage through dermatology texts and medical journals, often encountering truly abhorrent diseases. Rosacea didn't look so bad. But the more information I got, the clearer it was that while rosacea is not life-threatening, it should not be ignored. It is a progressive disease. Development is different from individual to individual. Environmental, life style and maybe genetic factors all play parts.

No one knows why some people develop rosacea and others don't. Researchers are starting to identify the risk factors. There is still no cure, but a significant percentage of rosacea sufferers manage the disease with the help of their dermatologists and by taking preventive measures to minimize flare-ups. Disease management is crucial to avoid the later stages of rosacea that can be disfiguring.

Ocular rosacea is another dimension of the disease that should be monitored. It was mentioned only casually in some sources; not mentioned at all in others. It wasn't until I got to the ophthalmology journals that I understood what a threat rosacea can be.

There are annoying symptoms like sties and dry, gritty eyes, but it can be more than that. Even the minor symptoms can affect your vision. Though it isn't common, it is possible for ocular rosacea to damage and even destroy your vision. This really got my attention.

Rosacea is increasing, probably because the baby boomers are reaching the age more apt to develop rosacea. Better diagnosis plays a part, too. Though rosacea has been around for a long time, it used to be harder to get a good diagnosis. People seem to be paying more attention to their appearance these days, too. Years ago as people got older, they didn't rush to the doctor if their skin started looking different. We are more apt to want to continue looking like Heather Locklear and Tom Cruise, even if we are over 50.

This book will serve as a resource for you in your effort to manage your disease. There are sections on the mechanics of what is happening under your skin. Other sections discuss common rosacea flare-up triggers and how to avoid them. There are sections on rosacea treatment. There is no cure, but there are drugs with a history of controlling the disease. I have included some alternative medical information, too. My recommendation is to use them in conjunction with conventional medical treatment, but the final decision is yours of course.

It turns out the ultimate responsibility for your life with rosacea rests with you. There are many ways to minimize its impact on your life and slow down its progress. They require some attention and discipline on your part, but ignoring your rosacea could result in something that isn't pretty. Literally.

Finally, I want to thank The National Rosacea Society for permission to use some of their materials in the book. They publish a quarterly newsletter that provides valuable information. They also conduct surveys, promote public education about rosacea and fund research. All their materials are free.

You can contact them at The National Rosacea Society, 800 South Northwest Highway Suite 200, Barrington, IL 60010. Their telephone number is 1-888-NO-BLUSH.

The e-mail address is rosaceas@aol.com. Their Web page is at http://www.rosacea.org.

CHAPTER 1
DEFINITION

OSACEA (ROSE-AY-SHAH) IS A COMMON inflammatory skin disease. It usually begins with a slight reddening of the cheeks, chin and nose, similar to a sunburn or blush that comes and goes. It then progresses to more frequent and prolonged facial reddening. Gradually, the redness becomes permanent. Tiny blood vessels on the cheeks, chin and nose become visible. Usually about this time, the skin erupts with pimple-like bumps. In the advanced stages, the nose can become enlarged and lumpy.

Rosacea may also affect the eyes. This is called ocular rosacea. The eyes may feel dry or gritty. Abnormal tear production may lead to conjunctivitis (called pink eye). Sties may develop on the edges of the eyelid. The eyelid edges may become inflamed and itchy. Lumps called chalazions may occur in the eyelid. Less commonly, the cornea may become inflamed and could be damaged.

While doctors are learning the mechanics of the disease (what is happening to the skin, underlying tissues and blood vessels), no one knows what causes it. Research has identified some things that trigger rosacea flare-ups, but there is no explanation of why these factors only affect some people.

Even though there is no cure for rosacea, there are treatments and lifestyle changes that can keep flare-ups to a minimum and prevent the disease from becoming worse.

Because the disease progresses slowly, many people don't recognize the symptoms and don't seek medical attention. It is important to see an ophthalmologist to determine if rosacea has affected your eyes, as well as seeing a dermatologist for diagnosis and treatment of the skin.

CLINICAL TERMS

The clinical terms for the symptoms of rosacea are:

blepharitis: inflammation of the eyelid edges

chalazion: clogged gland duct in the eyelid

conjunctivitis: inflammation of the thin, transparent lining of the eyelids and front of the eyeball

erythema: general redness of the skin

fibroplasia: excess of normal tissue caused by increased cell production

keratitis: infection or inflammation of the cornea

papules: small, red, solid pimples

pustules: pus-filled pimples

rhinophyma: swollen, red, bumpy nose

stye: an inflammation of an eyelash follicle
telangiectasia: tiny, red lines on the face

MECHANICS OF ROSACEA

Without trying to explain what causes these things to happen, we'll take a look at what medical science knows about what is going on with the visible skin, the underlying tissues, the capillaries in the skin and the eyes.

VISIBLE SKIN

Rosacea usually begins in fair-skinned people with a slight reddening of the facial skin. It looks like a blush, wind irritation or sunburn. The skin looks redder than usual across the cheeks and nose. The forehead and chin may also look redder, but the primary, affected areas are the cheeks and nose.

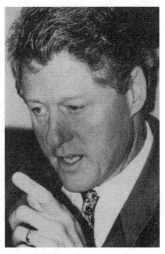

In the early stages of rosacea, the redness is temporary. As rosacea advances, the redness occurs more frequently and lasts longer.

Telangiectasia, or tiny red lines, appear on the face after the early stage of rosacea.

If rosacea is untreated, it can progress to the inflammatory stage when pimples appear. They can be solid (papules) or filled with pus (pustules). Unlike acne, blackheads (comedones) don't usually appear along with the pimples.

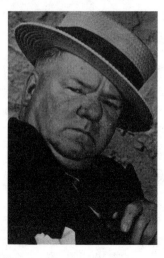

Usually the skin is dry, rather than oily, and it may itch or burn.

In advanced stages, the nose can become enlarged and lumpy. This is called rhinophyma. W.C. Fields is the poster boy for rhinophyma.

UNDERLYING TISSUES

Rosacea inflames the connective tissue of the dermis skin layer. The face may become swollen because of edema (excess fluid).

Fibroplasia (excess tissue) may create lumps under the skin. Rhinophyma is caused by enlarged sebaceous glands, excess tissue and fluid in the underlying tissue.

CAPILLARIES

Capillaries in the skin become dilated, or bigger around, and cause the facial skin to appear redder than normal. Dilated capillaries carry more blood. Blood is red. Some of the redness shows through the fair skin.

In the early stage of rosacea, the capillaries return to their normal size, so blood flow returns to normal and the skin returns to its normal color.

In later stages, the capillaries remain dilated. The redness doesn't go away, and the capillary walls become weak enough to allow blood to seep through. The blood that has seeped out shows up as telangiectasia, or tiny red lines on the face. The chapter on vascular aspects of rosacea examines this topic in greater detail.

EYES

Rosacea can affect the eyes, too. It usually starts with a grittiness or feeling as though you have something in your eye. Rosacea of the eyes can show up as conjunctivitis, blepharitis, sties and chalazions, too. We look at this in more detail in the chapter on ocular rosacea.

STEROID ROSACEA

There is a rosacea-like condition called steroid rosacea that is preventable and curable. It is caused by using strong steroid creams or ointments on the face.

After several weeks of using a topical steroid, the skin may become reddened and small bumps may appear. If the steroid cream is used for months or years, telangiectasia or spider veins may appear.

Because this condition is totally preventable by not using steroid creams for a long time, discuss possible alternative treatments if your doctor suggests steroid cream.

Steroid rosacea responds well to treatment. Topical steroid creams should be discontinued gradually, because an abrupt stop can make the condition worse. You can either apply the cream less frequently or change to a product that isn't as strong. Some times oral tetracycline is prescribed for a few months to clear up the signs of steroid rosacea. Laser treatment might be needed to repair the telangiectasia.

ROSACEA LYMPHEDEMA

This rosacea complication is rare. The central forehead, upper cheeks and area around the eyes progressively swell, usually symmetrically (the same on both sides of the face). Rosacea lymphedema is resistant to drug therapy, though systemic steroids may help. In severe cases, plastic surgery may be needed.

This is rare, and the swelling is very pronounced. We aren't talking about facial edema, which isn't rare. We are talking about really swollen.

CHAPTER 2
OCULAR ROSACEA

I F ROSACEA AFFECTS your eyes, you could have problems more serious than red skin, visible blood vessels, and lumps and bumps. While your face is important to your feeling of well-being, your eyes are more vital to your overall life.

Ocular rosacea is a set of inflammatory eye symptoms associated with rosacea. The symptoms include conjunctivitis, sties, chalazions, dry eyes or excessive tearing, crusty eyelids and inflammation of the cornea.

As with facial rosacea, there is no clear cause for ocular rosacea. Some theories that have been suggested, but not proven yet, are chronic staphylococcal infection, chronic inflammation of the Meibomian glands (glands that provide lubrication for the eyelids), *Demodex folliculorum* and vascular dysfunction. At least one study suggested all ocular rosacea problems involve the eyelids.

There aren't any firm numbers of how many rosacea sufferers experience ocular rosacea, but a 1969 study found as many as 58 percent have eye problems. If you know you have rosacea, you should probably see an ophthalmologist for an eye exam. Explain that you want to make sure rosacea has not affected your eyes, and ask for tips on minimizing possible eye damage.

Ocular rosacea often goes undiagnosed, according to a study done in 1996 at the Medical College of Georgia, Augusta. Patients with ocular rosacea often don't show signs of rosacea on the skin, and there is no one test for ocular rosacea. Interestingly, the same study found patients with less skin involvement showed more symptoms of ocular rosacea. So even if you don't have serious skin outbreaks, or maybe especially if you don't, you should pay special attention to your eyes.

Ocular rosacea often goes undiagnosed.

Trouble with your eyes may be the first clue you have rosacea. According to some reports, about 20 percent of rosacea sufferers develop eye symptoms before they show any facial symptoms. Sometimes ophthalmologists refer patients to dermatologists because they have seen signs of rosacea.

Awareness of the condition and its symptoms is your best defense against serious problems. The following information is not offered as a substitute for medical diagnosis and treatment, but as encouragement to seek medical advice if you recognize any of the signs of ocular rosacea.

Typically, ocular rosacea is treated with a combination of therapies tailored to the individual case. Therapy may include a combination of local and systemic treatments, as well as cleansing and tearing agents, all of which may be adjusted over time.

Before I did the research for this book, I mentioned my concerns about ocular rosacea to my eye doctor. He dismissed my concerns with the statement that he had never seen anyone go blind from rosacea. I'm currently searching for a new doctor. I am not comfortable with a care giver who has such a cavalier attitude toward my sight. I might feel differently if he had taken the time to explain how small the odds are, but he didn't even do that.

COMMON CONDITIONS OF OCULAR ROSACEA

The group of conditions that are grouped as ocular rosacea can affect the eyelids, the conjunctiva, the Meibomian glands and the cornea. Some of the conditions are mildly annoying, but others are sight-threatening.

The symptoms of the more potentially dangerous conditions are not the most dramatic, so please read this section carefully and consult your eye doctor if you recognize any of the symptoms. Your eye doctor is the only one who can determine if you have any of the listed conditions.

If you suspect you have one of the following conditions, it would be a good idea to stop wearing contact lenses until you see your doctor. Lenses can make some conditions worse.

STIES

A stye, or hordeolum, is an inflammation of an eyelash follicle on the edge of the eyelid. Each follicle has a gland that secretes oil to keep the eyelid soft and pliable. Bacteria can grow in the gland and then move to the follicle. A part of the eyelid edge will get red, sore and swollen.

The stye may come to a head, like a pimple. DO NOT squeeze it. That only spreads the infection. If the stye starts draining pus into your eye, see your eye doctor immediately.

Applying a warm, damp cloth to the eyelid four times a day for ten minutes may relieve the discomfort and reduce the swelling. Unless your eye doctor has given you other instructions, this is a good first line of attack.

If the stye doesn't go away in a couple days—or if a large area of your eyelid is swollen and you have a fever—consult your eye doctor to see if you need antibiotics.

If a gland deeper in the eyelid is involved, the condition is called an internal hordeolum. You may experience more discomfort with this kind of stye, and it usually doesn't go away by itself. Your eye doctor may have to cut into it to drain the pus. Internal hordeola often recur.

Sties are a common sign of ocular rosacea. In fact, a member of the dermatology department at Thomas Jefferson University Medical College in Philadelphia says, "Just about anybody who gets sties has rosacea or is eventually likely to develop the condition." If you have a history of developing them and haven't been diagnosed with ocular rosacea, you might want to ask your eye doctor to check your eyes carefully for other conditions associated with ocular rosacea.

The following illustration shows a stye on the bottom lid.

CHALAZIONS

A chalazion is a lump in the eyelid, but not in an eyelash follicle. The illustration above shows a chalazion on the upper lid. It develops from a clogged duct in one of the Meibomian glands in the eyelid. The lubricating oil that keeps your eyelids soft becomes trapped in a duct and gets hard.

From the outside of your eyelid, you may see a small bump. If you look on the inside of your eyelid, the chalazion may appear as either a red or gray mass.

Chalazions are not contagious or infected. Sometimes they respond to the warm, damp cloth treatment described for sties. Other times they just get bigger. Your eye doctor can remove them.

A steroid injection can shrink the chalazion. Sometimes it takes a month or more for the chalazion to disappear. One injection may do the trick, or you may need more than one. The injection stings, but isn't really painful.

Another option is to cut out, or excise, the chalazion. The incision is made on the inside of the eyelid, so you don't have a scar. The doctor will use a topical anesthetic, and you shouldn't feel anything. Recovery is generally a couple of days.

A study conducted several years ago found that 57 percent of people who had chalazions excised also had rosacea.

CONJUNCTIVITIS

Inflammation of the conjunctiva is called conjunctivitis or pink eye. The conjunctiva is the thin, transparent lining of the eyelids and front of the eyeball. Almost everyone I know has had it at least once. I remember one year when my daughter must have had it three times. It passed from child to child at her school.

There is no one cause of conjunctivitis. It may be a viral or bacterial infection; it may be a reaction to an allergy or irritant in the eye. Rosacea sufferers may develop conjunctivitis because of abnormal tear production.

Symptoms of conjunctivitis include eye swelling, redness, irritation and a discharge that can glue the eyelids together in the morning. Applying a warm, wet cloth is a safe way to unstick the gooey eyes. Don't be tough and just force your eyes open. You risk losing eye lashes and damaging the tender eyelid skin.

Treatment will likely be warm compresses and either eye drops or ointment.

Conjunctivitis can be highly contagious. Be sure to wash your hands frequently to avoid spreading any possible virus or bacteria. In addition to washing your hands before applying any medication, wash them after to avoid spreading the virus or bacteria to other parts of your own body.

BLEPHARITIS

This is an inflammation of the eyelid edges. The eyelids get red and irritated. You may have flakes of skin at the base of your eyelashes. The edges of the eyelids are often itchy. The eyes may feel dry and gritty. Symptoms may be worse after a night's sleep.

Blepharitis is often caused by staphylococcus infection and plugged glands in the eyelids.

The antibiotic doxycycline can be prescribed to kill off any bacteria; it may help unplug clogged glands, too. In addition to any medication your ophthalmologist gives you, warm compresses applied to the lids for ten to fifteen minutes twice a day for a month can help. Check with your eye doctor about cleaning the edges of your eyelids with a cotton swab dipped into diluted baby shampoo.

> *Tears are important to eye health.*

DRY EYE

Dry eye is more than annoying. It can be a real threat to eye health. The symptoms of dry eye include a gritty feeling in the eye. You may feel you have something in your eye, though you can't see anything there.

Dry eye is the result of abnormal tear production. Tears are important to eye health. The eye is constantly bathed by what is called the preocular tear film. The tear film serves several purposes. Without a healthy tear film, you don't get clear images to the retina. The tear film supplies nutrients and carries waste away from the cornea. It also protects the eye from bacteria.

Rosacea sufferers seem to have problems with maintaining a healthy tear film. One measure of tear film health is the tear break-up time (TBUT). This is the time it takes for a dry spot to show up on the eyeball. The average TBUT for the control group (folks without rosacea) in one study was 19.8 seconds; rosacea sufferers had an overall average TBUT of only 5.7 seconds before treatment. Rosacea sufferers with severe ocular symptoms had an average TBUT of 2.9 seconds.

An ophthalmologist may suggest you use artificial tears for good eye lubrication. Please note that artificial tears are different from products that promise to ease symptoms of eye redness.

You can suffer vision loss.

KERATITIS

This is a term used to describe infection or inflammation of the cornea (the portion of the eye that surrounds the pupil). Left untreated, keratitis can cause ulceration of the cornea, corneal vascularization and perforation—ultimately leading to vision loss.

Symptoms include sensitivity to light, blurred vision, eye pain, excess tearing and feeling as though you have something in your eyes. These symptoms may be signs of other eye conditions, but your ophthalmologist can perform a special eye exam to determine if your cornea is in trouble. If you normally wear contact lenses, you should not wear them until you see your eye doctor.

Medical treatment is important because if your cornea is damaged badly enough, you can suffer vision loss. Eye drops and ointments are commonly used to treat the condition. Early treatment is likely to be successful.

Early intervention if you suffer from keratitis is important because there is evidence that ocular rosacea patients are not good candidates for cornea transplants. Generally cornea transplants are among the most successful organ transplants—but not for ocular rosacea sufferers. Corneal vascularization and abnormal tearing tend to lead to cornea graft rejection.

DO NOT try to treat yourself. Non-prescription eye drops containing topical corticosteroids can make the condition worse.

Though keratitis is not common among rosacea sufferers, the possible consequences are serious enough to warrant paying special attention to your eyes.

TREATMENT OF OCULAR ROSACEA

Antibiotics seem to alleviate the symptoms of ocular rosacea. Studies showed tetracycline and doxycycline both worked effectively. One study found tetracycline worked faster, but doxycycline had fewer side effects.

A twelve-week study found that a course of doxycycline resulted in dramatic relief from ocular rosacea symptoms. Fourteen symptoms were graded, and 100% of study subjects reported reduction in seven of the symptoms. The other seven symptoms were reduced at rates ranging from 60% to 92%.

WEATHER AND OCULAR ROSACEA

Winter can be a tough time for patients with ocular rosacea. Cold winds are particularly drying and irritating to the eyes. If you have been diagnosed with ocular rosacea, try to stay out of the cold—especially cold winds. If you must go out, glasses or sunglasses will offer some eye protection.

CHAPTER 3
WHO DEVELOPS ROSACEA?

PRESIDENT **B**ILL **C**LINTON is among the fa mous folks who have the condition. W.C. Fields, the movie star from the 1930s, probably had rosacea. The American financier J.P. Morgan appears to have suffered from rosacea, too.

Winston Churchill, the former British prime minister, also had rosacea. Princess Diana is said to have experienced flare-ups of reddened skin. An article in the British medical journal *Lancet* said the Dutch artist Rembrandt's self portrait shows rosacea symptoms.

If it is any consolation, you are in illustrious company as a rosacea sufferer. Of course, it isn't only the rich and famous who develop rosacea.

The latest estimate is that 13,000,000 Americans suffer from rosacea. According to the National Rosacea Society, "...approximately one in every 20 Americans who will develop rosacea can probably answer 'yes' to one of the following questions:

"Are you over 30 years old?

"Do you flush or blush easily?

"Are you of Irish, English, Scottish or northern/eastern European descent?

"Do you have fair skin?

"Do you have family members who have been diagnosed with rosacea or experienced similar symptoms?

"Have you ever had a stye?

"Have you ever had a bad reaction to acne medication?"

The odds of developing rosacea are highest for people over 30. More than 40 percent are in their 30s or 40s. Another 44 percent develop the condition after the age of 50. People under the age of 30 only account for 13 percent of rosacea sufferers.

People who blush easily are more prone to develop rosacea.

People who flush or blush easily in their teenage and early-adult years appear to be more prone to develop rosacea. Tiny blood vessels in the face dilate when we blush or flush. While the reddening of the skin starts out as a response to physical exertion or emotional stress, someone with rosacea experiences increasingly frequent red skin.

A survey by the National Rosacea Society found 33 percent of rosacea sufferers have at least one parent of Irish descent. Another 27 percent reported at least one parent of English descent. Balkan, Lithuanian, Polish, Scandinavian, Scottish and Welsh ancestors also indicate a higher risk of rosacea than the rest of the population.

Fair skin is another indicator of being susceptible to rosacea. That shouldn't be surprising if you look at the ethnic groups who have higher risks of developing the condition. While rosacea is less common among people of Asian, Hispanic and African origin, they are not immune.

Heredity appears to be a factor in susceptibility for rosacea, too. The National Rosacea Society survey found "nearly 40 percent of rosacea patients surveyed could name a family member who had similar symptoms."

People who have a history of sties (eyelid infections) are more prone to developing rosacea. A stye may be a symptom of ocular rosacea, which can develop before the facial skin shows any signs of rosacea.

Sensitive skin is yet another sign of being at risk for rosacea. Bad reactions to acne medication is a particularly strong indication.

Did you notice that all these factors are beyond your control? You cannot pick your family, skin type or age. What you can do is understand your level of risk and watch for early signs of rosacea.

Early medical treatment of symptoms can prevent permanent skin and eye damage. If you are at high risk and notice reddening of the cheeks, pimples, visible tiny blood vessels, a gritty feeling or stinging in the eyes, sties or chalazions (lumps in the eyelids)—consult a dermatologist or ophthalmologist for diagnosis.

Do not try to treat yourself or wait for the symptoms to go away. If it is rosacea, it will probably get worse without proper treatment.

STATISTICS

Here are some numbers from a National Rosacea Society survey.

FAMILY

40% of rosacea sufferers have a family member with rosacea

27% have a parent with rosacea

18% have a brother or sister with rosacea

13% have a grandparent with rosacea

16% have an aunt or uncle with rosacea

11% have a son or daughter with rosacea

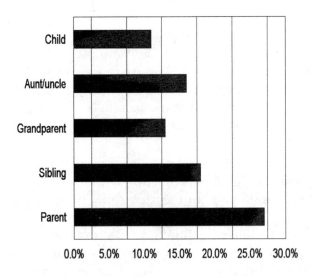

Family Members with Rosacea
National Rosacea Society survey

SKIN TYPE

more than 60% of rosacea sufferers have fair skin
35% have medium skin tones
less than 2% have dark skin

ANCESTRY

33% report one parent of Irish ancestry (U.S. Census figures report 15.6% of the general population has Irish roots).

26% report a parent of English ancestry (U.S. Census figures report 13% of the general population has English roots).

Rosacea Sufferer Ancestry
National Rosacea Society survey

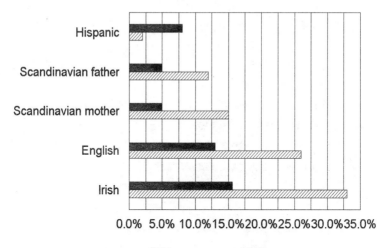

Nearly 15% report a mother of Scandinavian descent—12% report a father of Scandinavian descent (U.S. Census figures report 5% of the general population has Scandinavian roots).

Scottish, Welsh, Polish, Lithuanian and Balkan nationalities also reported higher rates of rosacea—folks with German, French, Italian, Greek and Russian backgrounds reported rates of rosacea that match their numbers in the general population.

While 8% of the U.S. population is Hispanic, only about 2% of the rosacea sufferers were Hispanic. There were few people of African or Asian ancestry among rosacea sufferers.

SYMPTOM STATISTICS

Here are more numbers from the National Rosacea Society showing symptom frequency and differences between how men and women typically experience rosacea.

Rosacea Symptoms Reported
National Rosacea Society survey

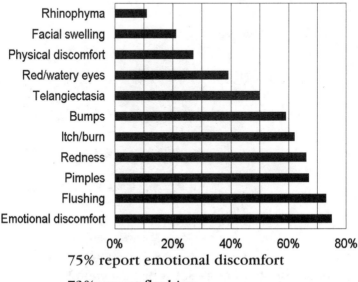

75% report emotional discomfort

73% report flushing

67% report pimples

66% report persistent redness

62% report itching or burning

59% report bumps

50% report telangiectasia

Nearly 40% report red or watery eyes

27% report at least occasional physical discomfort

21% report facial swelling

11% report an enlarged nose (rhino-phyma)

21% of men report rhinophyma

8% of women report rhinophyma

SYMPTOMS BY GENDER & LOCATION

49% of women report symptoms on the chin

20% of men report symptoms on the chin

87% of women report symptoms on the cheeks

68% of men report symptoms on the cheeks

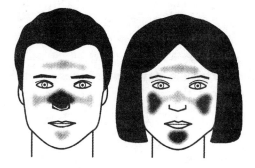

77% of women report symptoms on the nose

85% of men report symptoms on the nose

42% of women report symptoms on the forehead

41% of men report symptoms on the forehead

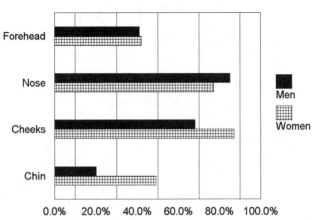

Symptom Location by Gender
National Rosacea Society survey

BLACKS AND ROSACEA

Though rosacea affects light-skinned people more frequently than other skin types, it is not unheard of among blacks. Flushing is not as prominent, probably because of the difference in skin pigmentation. Telangiectasia doesn't show up as often, either. In the advanced stages of rosacea, blacks develop papules, pustules and rhinophyma as fair-skinned sufferers do.

ROSACEA AMONG KOREANS

While rosacea is far more common among fair-skinned people, it is not unknown in Korea according to a study done at Inje University College of Medicine, Sanggye Paik Hospital in Seoul, South Korea. About one percent of the patients who visited the dermatology clinic were diagnosed with rosacea.

About two-thirds of the patients diagnosed were women. Korean patients showed symptom patterns different from those in England. Flushing and redness occurred at higher rates, but bumps, pimples and rhinophyma were less common. A theory is the Korean skin pigmentation may protect it from connective tissue degeneration caused by the sun. No one has a theory yet about why the Korean patients showed no symptoms of ocular rosacea.

CHAPTER 4
DIAGNOSIS

ARLY DIAGNOSIS OF ROSACEA is important, so you can start managing the condition. You might be able to do a self-diagnosis after seeing other people with rosacea and doing some reading, but you must see a health care provider, ideally a dermatologist, to be absolutely sure. You need to see an eye doctor for a diagnosis of ocular rosacea. And you must see a physician to get advice about medical treatment of rosacea. DO NOT think reading this book or talking to your cousin will give you the information you need for do-it-yourself treatment.

An accurate diagnosis is important regarding rosacea because the treatment for other conditions that rosacea may be confused with can make rosacea worse. For example, topical steroids are sometimes prescribed for seborrhoeic dermatitis. Steroids can intensify rosacea symptoms. In fact, long-term topical steroid use can bring on a form of rosacea.

Rosacea diagnosis is better than it used to be. In the past, people sometimes went years without a satisfactory answer to "what's going on with my face?" As the baby boomer generation enters the age group most susceptible to rosacea, they are streaming into doctors' offices. More general practitioners and family medicine providers recognize the condition nowadays. Whenever a condition or disease becomes more prevalent, professionals end up knowing more about it. Supply-and-demand drives medicine just as it drives the economy.

Even though non-dermatologists may provide a good diagnosis, a dermatologist is more likely to be familiar with the latest research about treating rosacea. Treatment may be complicated by a combination of conditions, too. Sometimes people have a form of dermatitis in addition to rosacea. It will probably take a good dermatologist to come up with a treatment plan that will manage each condition without making the other worse.

While the odds of your getting a good diagnosis are higher than they were 20 years ago, there are no guarantees.

These skin conditions might be confused with rosacea, because they present some of the same or similar symptoms.

ACNE VULGARIS

This is the acne usually found in teen-agers. Rosacea used to be commonly confused with it. In fact, for years rosacea was called adult acne. Acne vulgaris presents bumps and pimples, but it also usually involves blackheads (comedones in medical terms). Rosacea doesn't. The pimples in acne vulgaris stem from infection. Acne vulgaris doesn't cause telangiectasia, tiny visible blood vessels. Acne vulgaris pimples can appear anywhere on the face, while rosacea symptoms tend to be just in the central portion of the face. Also, flushing or blushing doesn't typically show up with acne vulgaris.

FOLLICULITIS

This superficial inflammation shows up as an itchy rash and pimples around hair follicles on the face, neck, legs and trunk. It can be a bacterial or fungal infection, and often stems from irritation to the follicles, like shaving or tight clothing.

PERIORAL DERMATITIS

This common skin condition appears as small red spots around the mouth (sometimes the spots are around the nose and on other areas of the face). The spots can itch and be tender. Young and middle-aged women are the likeliest sufferers. Men rarely suffer from perioral dermatitis.

There are a couple of theories of what causes perioral dermatitis. It might be a reaction to fluoridated steroid creams or prolonged use of topical corticosteroids (hydrocortisones). Premenstrual flare-ups are common.

Rosacea flare-ups present bumps and pimple-like papules, not red spots. Also, though rosacea skin may itch, the bumps and pimples usually don't.

CONTACT DERMATITIS

This is the name for any of the many allergic reactions to substances that come in contact with the skin—like poison ivy. It appears as an itching rash any place on the body. Contact dermatitis disappears after a short time and does not reappear unless you come in contact with the allergy-causing substance again.

SEBORRHOEIC DERMATITIS

This common, harmless, scaling rash sometime itches. Dandruff is seborrhoeic dermatitis of the scalp. Seborrhoeic dermatitis may appear on the eyebrows, eyelid edges, ears, near the nose and in the folds of the armpits and groin. Sometimes it shows up as round, scaling patches on the middle of the chest or back.

PITYROSPORUM FOLLICULITIS

This is another inflammation of hair follicles. A yeast called pityrosporum that is normally present on the skin causes an itching, acne-like condition when it multiplies in hair follicles. A rash usually appears on the upper back, shoulders and chest.

Pityrosporum folliculitis differs from rosacea because it appears in parts of the body other than the face.

LUPUS ERYTHEMATOSUS

This chronic inflammatory autoimmune disorder affects the skin, as well as joints and internal organs. It shows up as butterfly-shaped rash over the cheeks and bridge of the nose. While the location of symptoms matches rosacea, lupus erythematosus appears as macules (flat, red patches) rather than the bumps of rosacea.

PSORIASIS

Another chronic skin condition, psoriasis shouldn't be confused with rosacea. It takes many forms, but the most common is raised, red, round or oval scaling patches. These patches appear most often on the elbows, knees, scalp and lower back.

ECZEMA

This is a form of dermatitis that shows up as itchy, inflamed skin. Dry, thickened skin appears most often on the face, wrists, and inner creases of the elbows and knees. There may also be oozing blisters. Eczema and rosacea are not at all alike.

PROGNOSIS

Left untreated, rosacea usually becomes worse. Avoiding flare-up triggers may lessen or slow down the progress of the disease, but there is no evidence that rosacea ever "goes away" or even gets to one point and remains at that level.

There doesn't appear to be a clear connection between skin involvement and ocular rosacea progress. In fact, one study found that rosacea sufferers with ocular rosacea showed fewer skin-related symptoms.

With proper drug treatment and lifestyle changes to avoid flare-up triggers, the majority of rosacea sufferers manage to control the disease at a level they can live with.

Here is a breakdown of the generally-accepted stages of rosacea as it affects the skin.

STAGE 1

Erythema persists for hours and days. Telangiectasia becomes more visible on the nose, cheeks and the folds of skin between the nose and mouth. Skin may sting, burn or itch when fragrances, sunscreen and cosmetics are applied. Facial skin is particularly sensitive to chemical and physical stimulants.

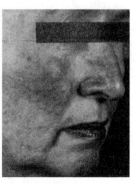

STAGE 2

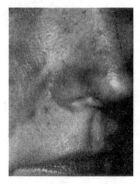

Papules and pustules appear and remain for weeks. Facial pores become larger and more visible. Papule/pustule attacks become more frequent. Rosacea may extend over the entire face, and even into the scalp if the patient is balding.

STAGE 3

A small percentage of rosacea sufferers develop nodules and tissue swelling, particularly on the cheeks and nose. The facial skin becomes thickened with large pores, resembling the peel of an orange.

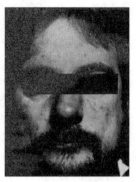

The sebaceous glands become extremely enlarged, forming dozens of papules on the cheeks, forehead, temples and nose.

CHAPTER 5
THEORIES OF CAUSES

THIS CHAPTER IS CALLED Theories of Causes because at this time, medical science hasn't come up with a definite cause for rosacea. There have been theories for many years, but no agreement on any of them. Before a theory can be accepted as a definitive cause, research has to find the same answers over and over again. So far that hasn't happened.

It may turn out that one or more of the theories is right, but the results weren't duplicated because of yet unknown factors. As researchers learn more, they should be able to identify more of the factors involved, and figure out which are causes and which are effects.

OLD THEORIES

Let's start with ideas about rosacea that have not stood the test of time. On the whole, they appear now as judgmental opinions rather than scientific theories.

PERSONALITY DISORDERS

A book written in 1953 says:

> The outstanding characteristic of rosacea patients is a level of self-esteem so abnormally [low] that it is constantly threatened by what to others are everyday events. The anxious dependence on the good opinion of others, the compulsive desire to please, the constant fear of attracting attention, indicate the existence of unreasonably strong feelings of inferiority, guilt and shame.

These same learned authors discuss blushing, too. According to them, "Blushing is incompatible with complete innocence and modesty. It occurs most often and most typically in individuals in whom conflict between morality and sexual impulses are most common and severe and at phases of life when these conflicts are especially acute."

I don't know about you, but I'm glad I didn't have to consult them about medical problems.

ALCOHOL ABUSE

For many years, flushed cheeks and an enlarged nose were seen only as signs of alcoholism. Men with rhinophyma (a bulbous, lumpy nose from tissue build-up) were assumed to be drunks. W.C. Fields always seemed to be half-lit in his movies. It even became a quick way to portray an unsavory character in both books and movies.

A Web page sponsored by a well-known medical figure states rosacea is associated with alcoholism. Old ideas die hard. I want to stress that current research clearly demonstrates there is no causal connection between alcoholism and rosacea.

Alcohol can trigger a rosacea flare-up, but there is no evidence that alcohol causes rosacea. People who don't drink at all, let alone to excess, still develop rosacea.

CURRENTTHEORIES

Our great-grandchildren may look back on the current theories about rosacea and find them as absurd as we find the older theories. That happens quite often in science. Right now, though, researchers continue to explore the following theories.

DEMODEX FOLLICULORUM

This tiny (0.3 mm long) parasite lives in hair follicles. *Demodex folliculorum* is found most frequently on the face, scalp and upper chest. There have been quite a few studies about the connection between *Demodex folliculorum* and rosacea. A theory was that mite infestations caused rosacea papules and pustules.

Don't think about this too long, it will only make you feel creepy. Try to remember that it is perfectly normal to have little critters living in your body. Most of them are there to maintain some kind of balance and don't harm us. Especially if we don't think about them! Whatever you do, don't start scrubbing your face to get rid of the mites. They live deep in the skin. Scrubbing is never a good idea for rosacea sufferers.

Many people without skin problems also have *Demodex folliculorum*, so researchers looked at the density of the mites rather than the mites just being there. They wanted to find out if a concentration of *Demodex folliculorum* was the cause of rosacea.

One study found the highest concentration of mites on the cheeks. Rosacea sufferers had more than twice the *Demodex folliculorum* infestation than people without rosacea.

When they examined the concentration of mites, they found almost two and a half times as many *Demodex folliculorum* in a square centimeter of skin of rosacea sufferers compared to the control group. Rosacea sufferers with papules and pustules showed the greatest difference from the control group. Some studies confirm the higher concentration of *Demodex folliculorum* in the skin of rosacea sufferers, but at least one other study couldn't confirm those findings.

The biggest question though is whether the mites are contributing factors to rosacea or a result of the disease. The arguments for being a cause include:

Immune agents the body releases—to combat the *Demodex folliculorum*—damage skin tissue and create papules and pustules.

Demodex folliculorum clog the follicles they live in.

On the other hand, *Demodex folliculorum* may find a comfortable environment in skin that is already damaged by swelling and leaky capillaries.

This is another example of not knowing for sure which came first. We encounter this situation frequently when looking at rosacea's symptoms and suspected causes. Again, further research is needed.

HELICOBACTER PYLORI

Helicobacter pylori (Hp) was recently discovered to be the cause of many stomach ulcers. It has shown up in rosacea sufferers' gastric juices, which leads some researchers to believe it may be a contributing factor to or cause of rosacea.

This theory is strengthened by the observation that certain foods trigger rosacea flare-ups. A study reported that rosacea sufferers have more indigestion than the general public. A study reported that people suffer from both peptic ulcer and rosacea flare-ups more frequently in the spring. Someone else found the rate of Hp infection was higher in rosacea sufferers than among the general public. Some drug therapies have eradicated Hp in rosacea sufferers, and those patients showed no signs of either ulcers or rosacea.

People suffer from rosacea flare-ups more frequently in the spring.

All this evidence made it look like Hp and rosacea were intertwined. Some doctors began to treat rosacea sufferers for Hp. In many cases, both Hp and rosacea disappeared after treatment.

In one study, though, rosacea symptoms reappeared months later in all the research subjects even though Hp didn't reappear. Two different studies performed specifically to determine the relationship between *Helicobacter pylori* and rosacea found no unusual appearance of Hp in rosacea sufferers. Rosacea sufferers were just as likely to have Hp infection as anyone else. In fact, one subset of research subjects with rosacea had a smaller than average percentage of Hp infection.

An article on *Helicobacter pylori* mentioned that Hp infection can cause histamine release. Since histamines can cause blood vessel dilation, maybe that is the link between Hp and rosacea. More research may yield the answer.

Overall, more research is needed to definitively prove or disprove the *Helicobacter pylori*/rosacea connection. The conflicting results and conclusions leave the question unanswered.

CAPILLARIES & UNDERLYING TISSUES

When researchers examine the capillaries and underlying skin tissue of patients suffering from advanced stages of rosacea, they usually find both the capillaries and skin tissue are damaged.

For awhile there was a theory that damaged underlying tissue didn't provide proper support for the capillaries in the dermis layer of the skin. Without good support, the capillaries suffered their own damage that led to blood and other fluids leaking from the tiny blood vessels.

Recent research, however, found that capillary damage showed up earlier than tissue damage, so it appears that fluids leaking from capillaries may cause the tissue damage. More research is needed before we'll know for sure.

VIDEO DISPLAY TERMINALS

A study in Norway in the 1980s reported a higher incidence of rosacea among women who worked in front of video display terminals, or computer monitors. When a survey was conducted here in the United States, the results were not conclusive. It discovered that there were women who worked in front of computer monitors who had rosacea, but there was no controlled research to determine if and how the monitors affected rosacea.

Obviously, computers cannot cause rosacea because it has been around far longer than computers. It might be possible that radiation from the monitor affects the rosacea sufferers' sensitive skin. I couldn't find any follow-up surveys or any research studies.

If you think it might be a factor in your rosacea, talk to a knowledgeable computer sales person about radiation shields that go over the front of the monitor.

NOT QUITE A THEORY

Rosacea exhibits some of the same patterns as an allergy: flushed skin, swelling and itching. Certain foods trigger flare-ups that could be viewed as mild allergic reactions. Many foods that are well-known allergens for many people appear on the list of common flare-up triggers.

Personally, I would like to see research to determine possible connections among edema, capillary dilation and damage, histamine production, migraine headaches and indigestion. I came across studies that mentioned histamines, migraines and indigestion almost as coincidences or after-thoughts. They look worth investigating to me, but nobody has asked me for my opinion yet. It's funny how often that happens. (The Secretary General of the United Nations hasn't called me to find out how to solve world problems, either.)

The final answer about the cause of rosacea is probably more complicated than just an allergy, because there are other factors—like weather and exercise—that can also trigger flare-ups.

THE BOTTOM LINE

Since medical science doesn't know the cause of rosacea, there is no cure. Neither is there any known way to prevent developing it. The best we can do is deal with the symptoms.

Dealing with symptoms means avoiding triggers and treating the skin well to minimize damage from the flare-up episodes.

CHAPTER 6
SKIN

L ET'S TAKE A LOOK at skin to better under
stand what is happening when you have a
rosacea flare-up. A brief and simple explanation of skin function and structure may
remove some of the mystery of how your skin's
appearance can dramatically change.

Did you know the skin is considered one of
your organs? Actually, it is the largest organ in
your body. On average, an adult's skin weighs
between six and seven pounds. That's twice as
big as the average adult brain.

Not only is it big, it is important. In addition
to keeping your insides in, your skin protects
your internal organs from harmful substances.
The skin has chemicals and good bacteria that
protect the body from micro-organisms.

The skin pigment melanin protects the body
from ultraviolet radiation. When your skin is exposed to bright sun light, it produces more
melanin in an attempt to keep the ultraviolet
radiation from internal organs. We call that process getting a tan. Some people think a tan makes

them look healthier, but in reality it is a sign of the body's struggle to protect itself from damaging radiation.

The skin also helps regulate your body temperature. The body is designed to operate within a pretty small range of temperatures. If it gets either too hot or too cold, things stop working right.

One of the skin layers contains fat that acts as insulation. Just like a blanket, it prevents the internal body heat from escaping through the skin.

Blood vessels close to the surface of the skin also regulate the body's temperature. When a portion of the body is exposed to cold temperature, less blood flows to the area to decrease heat loss. If normal blood flow continued through the chilled area, the blood's temperature would drop and then cool other parts of the body.

When your body starts to get too warm, either from internal heat like a fever or external heat, blood vessels dilate to increase heat loss. As more blood flows close to the skin's surface, the rate of heat transfer from the hot body to the cooler air increases. That keeps the internal organs from getting too hot.

The skin also contains sweat glands that help in body temperature regulation. Sweat glands produce moisture that cools the body as it evaporates on the skin. Evaporation uses up heat. That's why splashing your skin with water makes you feel cooler, even if the water isn't cold.

The skin also works like a factory. It produces vitamin D from sunlight. The body makes a compound from cholesterol and stores it in the skin. The sun acts on that compound to create vitamin D, which is then stored in the liver. Vitamin D helps the body absorb calcium, which is a vital nutrient for strong bones.

The skin also serves as sense organ—transmitting messages of heat, cold, pressure, pain, tickle and itch to the brain.

There is no evidence that rosacea prevents your skin from performing any of its important functions. It seems there are no secondary health threats from rosacea. Your skin will still regulate temperature, protect you from infections and produce vitamin D even if rosacea reaches its advanced stages.

ANATOMY OF SKIN

The skin is made up of three main layers. From the outside they are the epidermis, the dermis and the subcutaneous layer or tissue.

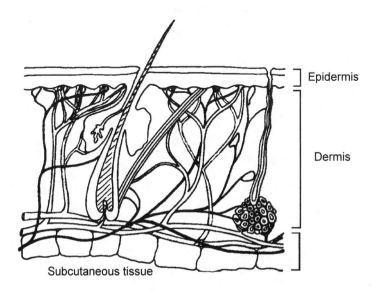

Epidermis

Dermis

Subcutaneous tissue

EPIDERMIS

The epidermis is the top layer of skin. It, in turn, has sub-layers. The deepest layer of the epidermis, called the basal layer, is where skin cells form. Melanin is produced in the basal layer, too.

The skin cells move up through the prickle cell layer (don't you wonder sometimes how scientists come up with names?). This layer also contains Langerhans cells that can attack organisms that have entered the skin.

Next is the granular layer. Here the cells get thicker because keratin starts forming here. Keratin is the protein that makes the outermost layer of skin waterproof.

Finally we get to the skin you can see. It is called the horny layer or stratum corneum. By the time the cells reach the surface, they are dead and ready to be discarded. The trip up from the basal layer to the surface of the skin takes anywhere from eight to eleven weeks. The stratum corneum cells are tightly interlocked, like bricks in a wall, to keep body fluids in and harmful substances out.

That's a lot of activity in the thin, outermost layer of skin. And, somehow, a healthy epidermis knows how to balance new cell production with dead cell loss. It only makes as many new cells as it needs to replace the dead cells that fall or are scraped off every day.

DERMIS

The living layer of skin is the dermis. The second main layer of the skin, it lies directly below the epidermis. The dermis serves as the support system for the epidermis. It supplies nutrients to that upper main layer of skin.

The capillaries that are so important to rosacea are in the dermis layer. In addition to feeding
both the dermis and epidermis (the epidermis
doesn't contain its own blood supply), the capillaries help regulate body temperature. See the
chapter on vascular aspects of rosacea for more
information about capillaries.

The dermis contains connective tissue that
gives the skin strength and elasticity. It also has
immune cells that fight any invaders that make
it through the epidermis. Sweat glands—that col-
lect water and waste products from blood vessels
and release them to skin pores—are in the dermis. The dermis is also where the hair roots are.
Hair grows in the dermis; by the time you can
see hair coming through the epidermis it is dead.
Nerves that transmit pain, temperature and
touch messages to the brain are in the dermis.

SUBCUTANEOUS TISSUE

The dermis is attached to muscles and bones by
the subcutaneous tissue. Subcutaneous tissue
provides an insulating layer to help regulate
body temperature. It also acts as a shock ab-
sorber, cushioning delicate organs under the
skin from all the bumps and jars of daily life.
The thickness of the subcutaneous tissue varies
throughout the body. It is thicker on the but-
tocks and abdomen than on the back of the hand
(I'm certainly grateful for that!).

PHOTO-DAMAGED SKIN

Skin normally suffers damage as we age. Just
look at a baby and then in the mirror to see a
dramatic example. Older skin has fewer capillaries and elastic fibers, has less collagen and is

thinner. Photo-damaged skin shows all the signs of older skin—earlier and more dramatically.

Any connection between photo- (light) damaged skin and rosacea is unclear, but since rosacea sufferers have damaged capillaries and underlying skin tissue, it makes sense to minimize future injury to the skin by wearing sun screen.

LYMPHATIC SYSTEM

The lymphatic system, a specialized part of the circulatory system, maintains the body's fluid balance and helps fight infection. Lymph vessels run throughout the body, roughly parallel to veins and arteries. They lie in the dermis next to the capillaries, too.

Lymph vessels carry a fluid called lymph that comes from both the blood and tissue fluids. The space around cells is call interstitial space. Plasma, the watery part of blood, filters out of capillaries into the interstitial space where cells absorb it. When the body is doing everything right, any fluid left over—after the cells have filled up—is reabsorbed by the lymph vessels. If the lymph vessels don't carry away the excess fluid, the fluid left over causes edema (swelling). Massive edema damages or even kills tissues.

EFFECTS OF ROSACEA ON SKIN

Some effects of rosacea on the skin are unclear. In some cases, there is disagreement among medical researchers about which are the causes and which are the effects of skin damage.

Underlying skin tissue appears to be damaged in rosacea sufferers. This damage may be the effect of capillaries releasing too much fluid into the interstitial space around cells. It may be the effect of the lymph vessels not recapturing enough of the fluid.

The abnormal tissue growth (fibroplasia) in the later stages of rosacea may be the result of edema, or swelling, caused by the excess interstitial fluid. Fibroplasia may be caused by the capillaries leaking a substance known as blood coagulation factor XIII. Yet another theory is that the swelling caused by papules and pustules may cause fibroplasia.

Underlying skin tissue appears to be damaged in rosacea sufferers.

The flushing rosacea sufferers experience may be the effect of an inflammation of underlying tissue which triggers an immune response that makes the dermis thinner. Some researchers believe the capillaries become damaged from early episodes of flushing—caused by dilated capillaries—and are then unable to return to their normal size. Just as a balloon becomes less flexible after you blow it up several times, and can't return to its original shape.

Some researchers refer to telangiectasia as leaky capillaries, while others call them enlarged capillaries. The capillaries may be visible because the dermis layer of skin becomes thinner.

It would appear we are a long way from understanding this disease. Until medical research makes some major breakthrough, we are left to deal with the symptoms as best we can.

CHAPTER 7
VASCULAR SYSTEM AND ROSACEA

Rosacea is generally thought of as a skin disease. The effects of rosacea appear on the skin, so it seems natural to call it a skin disease. It may not be that simple (not that anything about rosacea is simple!).

If we look beneath the skin, we see blood vessels are involved in rosacea. The reddening of the skin is caused by blood vessels dilating. The spider veins or telangiectasia that show up in later stages of rosacea are signs of damaged capillaries.

A study in Sweden found female rosacea sufferers between the ages of 50 and 60 were more apt to experience migraine headaches than women without rosacea. Thirteen percent of the general population suffer from migraine, but 27% of women with rosacea (between 50 and 60 years) have migraines. Researchers don't know why, but theorize it might be connected to changes in how blood vessels react to hormone changes after menopause.

This theory supports looking at rosacea as a vascular disease that affects the skin, rather than a skin disease. While treating symptoms that appear on the skin is important, improving vascular health may be even more important in the long run.

Let's take a look at the vascular system to better understand what is happening under the skin.

VASCULAR SYSTEM

Blood circulates through the body, feeding tissues and carrying away waste via the vascular system. A closed-system network of blood vessels allows blood to move from the heart to every cell in the body and back to the heart.

Oxygen-rich blood is pumped out of the heart through arteries. Arteries are relatively large vessels that carry the blood throughout the body. They are the thickest, toughest and most flexible of the blood vessels so they can handle the pressure from blood being pumped by the heart. They branch off to tiny capillaries, where tissue "feeding" and waste removal actually take place. Capillaries then connect to veins. Veins carry the blood back to the heart, which sends blood to the lungs to pick up more oxygen. The larger veins—in the arms and legs—have one-way valves that keep blood from moving backwards. This is important because blood is frequently flowing against gravity to get back to the heart. Then the whole cycle begins again.

CAPILLARIES

We are primarily interested in the capillaries, because they are involved with rosacea symptoms.

These blood vessels are incredibly small. One source said a capillary is 1/50 as thick as a baby's hair. Some capillaries are so small, red blood cells pass through one cell at a time. The walls of a capillary are only one cell thick. That makes it easy to understand how this fragile structure can become damaged. What is more amazing is how healthy capillaries avoid being damaged!

A capillary is 1/50 as thick as a baby's hair.

Capillaries are able to deliver oxygen to tissue because their walls are so thin. Red blood cells traveling through arteries carry the oxygen from the lungs and then release it through the capillaries. The oxygen feeds the tissues. Carbon dioxide passes from tissue cells through the capillary walls into the red blood cells. The red blood cells then travel through the veins back to the lungs, where the carbon dioxide is "unloaded," and we exhale it.

Capillaries also help regulate the body's temperature. When the body is overheated, the blood gets hotter. When capillaries receive that hot blood, they dilate to release the excess heat to the surrounding tissue. The skin gets redder, or flushed.

CAPILLARIES AND ROSACEA

When a rosacea sufferer flushes, capillaries dilate or become bigger around (think of blowing up a balloon). The dilated capillary allows more blood to flow, and the skin gets pinker. Under perfect conditions, the capillary is elastic enough to handle the stress of being stretched and returns to its normal size when the flush is over.

For reasons medical science hasn't fully explained, rosacea sufferers' capillaries become less elastic and don't return to normal size. Without preventive medicine and/or lifestyle changes, rosacea sufferers tend to flush more easily and frequently as the disease progresses.

After awhile, it isn't completely clear if the flushing is a cause or sign of damaged capillaries. It makes sense that frequent stretching of the capillaries would damage them, but then they would stretch more easily once they are damaged.

In addition to their own elastic nature, capillaries are supported by the connective tissue that surrounds them. There was a theory that the connective tissue under the skin was damaged and didn't provide proper support for the capillaries, so they deteriorated. Another theory was that leaky capillaries damaged the connective tissue.

It appears now that capillary deterioration occurs before the connective tissue damage, so the capillaries are the culprit rather than the victim. The capillary deterioration may be a result of environmental factors—primarily damage from ultraviolet rays of the sun. This would fit with the fact that people with fair skin are more apt to develop rosacea.

When capillaries are more severely damaged, rosacea sufferers experience more than a flush. Telangiectasia (visible capillaries) appear as tiny red lines on the face. At this point the capillaries are so badly damaged, they are leaking blood through their thin walls.

Until medical science figures exactly how and why the capillaries of rosacea sufferers are more likely to become damaged, we are left with the best defense of avoiding the flush reaction that seems to cause the damage.

FLUSHING

One sign of susceptibility to rosacea is easily blushing or flushing. The most common symptom of rosacea is a flushed look on the cheeks and nose (less frequently on the chin).

Blushing/flushing can be caused by emotional or physical factors. We tend to call it blushing when embarrassment is the trigger. I'll use the word flush, to save some keystrokes.

Emotional or physical stress sends a message to the blood vessels to dilate, or get a bit bigger around, to bring more blood to the muscles. This would be helpful if you were about to run away from an enemy or stand there and fight, because the extra blood fuels the muscles.

In addition to the emotional or physical stress a person notices, rosacea sufferers seem to experience stresses they don't notice—until the flush appears. For reasons we don't understand yet, rosacea sufferers flush more easily and frequently than the rest of the population.

There are several types of flushings. By recognizing the different types, you may be able to avoid them. We'll discuss them further in the chapter on managing rosacea.

Cold weather flushing occurs when you enter a warm room or building after being out in the cold.

The body is trying to quickly restore/balance its temperature.

Heavy meal flushing is the result of eating a heavy meal (who would have guessed, eh?).

Heavy meals need increased blood flow for digestion.

Sugar/carbohydrate flushing comes from a rapid influx of sugar into the blood stream. This dilates blood vessels, dispersing the energy quickly through the system.

Steroid flushing is a thinning of the skin and telangiectasia from prolonged use of steroid creams.

Adrenalin flushing is caused by an adrenalin rush in response to stress. The hormone adrenalin causes the blood vessels in the face—and elsewhere—to dilate, readying the body for action.

Exercise flushing is the result of the cardiovascular system pumping blood harder and faster.

Cigarette flushing occurs because smoking creates free radicals that damage capillaries.

Hot shower/bath flushing is caused by the stimulation of hot water on the skin's surface.

Alcohol flushing occurs because alcohol is a diuretic and forces water out of cells. A dehydrated body is more prone to flushing. The blood vessels also dilate because alcohol is metabolized quickly, much the same as sugar.

Flushing can also be caused by sun exposure, wind exposure, histamine production, allergic reaction, abrasive skin products and laughter.

CHAPTER 8
ROSACEA MANAGEMENT

ROSACEA IS A CHRONIC condition with no known cure. All the evidence says once you have rosacea, you have rosacea. It is important to understand that—as hard as it might be to accept. Most of us are uncomfortable with the whole idea of incurable. We grew up during the most dramatic times in medical history.

Medical science has come up with wonder cures for dozens, if not hundreds, of conditions that have plagued human beings since the beginning of time. Millions and millions of dollars are spent each year on medical research. Pharmaceutical and bio-tech companies are some of the hottest companies around.

"If we can put a man on the moon, why can't we cure rosacea?"

There are probably many reasons. Though the estimates are that about 13 million Americans suffer from rosacea, those numbers weren't as large in the past. There weren't as many people with rosacea, so there wasn't a sizable population looking for relief. Reliable diagnosis of rosacea wasn't the norm until recently. Lots of people didn't even know they had rosacea, so they weren't asking for a cure.

The biggest reason might be that research money only goes so far. There is a limit on the number of research projects that will receive funding each year. Since rosacea isn't life-threatening, arguments for research money might be hard to make.

That said, as the size of the rosacea population grows, demands for a cure are bound to increase. Even non-life-threatening conditions can present enough pressure for research if they affect a large enough group of people.

Before scientists can find a cure, they will have to determine the cause or causes of rosacea. As the chapter on causes showed, current research is far from consensus on this issue.

Rosacea sufferers themselves may be able to assist in determining causes by tracking their triggers and responding to surveys about rosacea.

Between 85 and 90 percent of people state that medical treatment reduced their symptoms.

So while the bad news is that there is no cure, the good news is that there are plenty of things you can do to keep rosacea flare-ups to a minimum. National Rosacea Society surveys report between 85 and 90 percent of people state that medical treatment reduced their symptoms.

The most important thing is to stay on any

medication your dermatologist prescribes. Most of the research shows medication should be ongoing—not just used during a flare-up. The purpose of the medication isn't to clear up flare-ups, but to prevent them. Flare-ups are not only unpleasant, but may be doing further damage to the skin tissue and blood vessels.

The temptation may be to discontinue medication if you don't see any signs of rosacea. Unless your dermatologist tells you to discontinue, don't do it. If the doctor does tell you to discontinue, you might ask why. Research shows flare-ups tend to recur when you stop taking medication.

There may be a legitimate reason for discontinuing medication, but it is a good idea to find out what it is. An involved, informed patient usually gets better medical care.

In addition to prescribed medicines, there are things you can do for yourself to keep flare-ups to a minimum. Notice I said "in addition" to medicines. The following suggestions are not a substitute for a doctor's regimen of care. You still need to see a dermatologist and follow those orders. If the doctor's advice differs from anything in this book, discuss what you want to do. These are general suggestions, and your rosacea or other health conditions may require other care.

DEALING WITH HEAT

Being overheated can bring on flushing. As best you can, avoid getting hot. If you can be in air conditioning during hot weather—do it. If you don't have that option, drink plenty of cold liquids or chew on ice chips to stay cool. You could also spray water on your face or keep a cool, damp cloth at hand.

When you exercise, be sure to drink cold liquids or chew on ice chips. Putting a cool, damp towel around your neck will help keep you from overheating. Avoid outdoor exercise during the warmest hours of the day—typically from 10:00 in the morning until 2:00 in the afternoon.

Do your outdoor chores in the early morning. If you have to be outside when it is hot, slow down. Rushing will add to the intensity of any flushing. Wear a hat when you go out in hot weather, even if you don't the rest of the time. Women, buy a simple, inexpensive straw hat and dress it up with scarves, ribbons, silk flowers, pins—have fun with it. Who knows, as the population of rosacea sufferers grows, we may bring hats back into fashion.

Fix simple meals on hot days, so you don't spend time over a hot stove. Use your rosacea as a valid excuse to get your teenaged children out there mowing the lawn and washing the car. It will be good for them.

DEALING WITH COLD

Being cold can also bring on flushing (sometimes you just can't win). If you must be outdoors during cold weather, wrap a scarf around the lower part of your face to shield it from the cold and wind. When it is very cold, a ski mask offers better protection. (Just be careful about going into a bank!)

Hire a kid, if you don't have one handy, to shovel the snow off the sidewalk. Rosacea or not, most men in their 50s and 60s shouldn't be shoveling snow anyway. Every year, seemingly healthy men drop dead from heart attacks while shoveling snow.

If your face does get cold, don't try the old trick of slapping your cheeks to warm them. Don't even rub them roughly. Your skin and blood vessels are more fragile than normal, and such rough treatment may further damage them.

It is a good idea to avoid sudden temperature changes, too. So don't keep your house too hot in the winter. Coming into a hot house from the outside cold will certainly make you flush.

EXERCISE TIPS

You may need to modify your exercise program if it includes strenuous activities. Working up a good sweat may bring on a pleasant endorphin high, but it isn't good for your rosacea.

A high-intensity workout is likely to bring on flushing. Shorter and more frequent lower-intensity activities can be just as effective, without triggering a flush. Instead of jogging, try walking to burn off calories. If chlorine doesn't bother your skin badly, swimming is a good exercise for the cardiovascular system. Working with free weights can build strength and stamina without working up a sweat.

The days of "no pain, no gain" are gone.

If you like to bicycle, take it leisurely rather than trying to emulate the Tour de France. The days of "no pain, no gain" are gone. Even Jane Fonda is doing kinder, gentler exercises these days. Even if you are among the younger rosacea sufferers, you might want to check out exercises for older people. They are likely to be less strenuous.

If you exercise outdoors, avoid the mid-afternoon when the sun is the hottest. Keep your inside exercise area well-ventilated to avoid overheating. Drinking cool water, chewing on ice chips, draping a cool, damp towel around your neck, and spraying your face with cool water will help keep flushing to a minimum.

CIGARETTES

You won't be surprised to hear that rosacea sufferers who smoke should stop. Cigarette smoking destroys vitamin C—a nutrient vital to the health of skin. Smoking creates free radicals that damage capillaries. It also robs the skin of oxygen, which can be a contributing factor to telangiectasia. If anyone has done a study about second-hand smoke and rosacea, it didn't show up in any of the major journals.

MENOPAUSE AND ROSACEA

Since rosacea commonly occurs in the 50s, women stand a good chance of going through menopause with rosacea. The flushing that some women experience with menopause may be as damaging as all the other kinds of flushing.

Hormone replacement therapy (HRT) may help relieve the flushing. HRT is a complicated issue, though. It is about more than flushing. It is about breast cancer, heart disease, osteoporosis and other health issues. After discussing the pros and cons of HRT with your doctor, you are the only one who can decide if you want to take hormones.

SKIN CARE

Follow the suggestions in the chapter on skin care. Remember to be gentle to your skin. Avoid really hot baths, showers and saunas. Watch carefully for products that irritate your skin.

MEDICAL CONDITIONS

A simple cold with its coughing may bring on a rosacea flare-up. Use cough drops or syrups to keep coughing to a minimum. Of course, you should to your doctor about a persistent cough.

The fever that accompanies the flu can also trigger a flare-up. Aspirin is the usual drug to bring fever under control (never give aspirin to a child with a fever without consulting your doctor), but if you are sensitive to salicylate, talk to your doctor about alternate medicines.

High blood pressure can cause flare-ups. If you think you have high blood pressure, be sure to talk to your doctor about bringing it under control. If you already know you have it, rosacea is another reason (as if you needed another) to take your high blood pressure medication.

DRUGS

Vasodilator drugs, prescribed for some cardio-vascular diseases, have been known to cause flushing. If you are taking drugs for cardiovascular disease, DON'T stop taking them to avoid flushing. Talk to your doctor about what you can do to minimize the flushing.

Topical steroids can make rosacea worse, or even bring on what is called steroid-induced rosacea. If your doctor prescribes topical steroids, see if there is a another medication you could use. If there isn't, ask your doctor for suggestions to avoid making your rosacea worse.

FOOD AND BEVERAGES

See the chapter on food for more information about flare-up triggers. We both know you are apt to use the food trigger list to avoid your mother-in-law's eggplant casserole if you don't like eggplant. And you are probably going to forget you even saw chocolate on the list if it is your favorite treat.

Reading the list of foods and ingredients that can trigger rosacea flare-ups may seem daunting. There are conflicts between foods that are good for and those that might cause a flare-up. This is not an exact science. Obviously, you cannot follow all the tips in this book. There are just too many of them, and they are contradictory. You are going to have to do some research testing on yourself to see just what your triggers are.

ROSACEA DIARY CHECKLIST

The National Rosacea Society has made up a diary checklist to help rosacea sufferers figure out which foods and activities trigger flare-ups. They gave me permission to include a copy of it in this book. I had to adapt it to make it fit on these smaller pages, so it isn't as pretty as their original. You will find it at the back of the book in the Appendix.

By filling in the checklist at the end of the day, you keep track of what you were exposed to that day. You also make note of your skin's condition that day. After doing this for a few cycles of rosacea flare-ups, you may be able to identify possible triggers.

It is important to have records of days both when you experience flare-ups and when you don't. You need consecutive daily records, too—not scattered days when you happen to think of filling in the checklist.

Records from days without flare-ups serve as your baseline. Records from days with flare-ups and the days before flare-ups will show what is different from the baseline time. Activities and foods that show up on the checklist before a flare-up are possible triggers. Some triggers work faster than others. One day in the bright sun may bring on a flare-up that day. On the other hand, it make take several days of increased stress to cause a flare-up.

You should keep records for awhile before you start changing your routine. Without a sturdy baseline, you can't be sure of what you need to change.

Once you have a set of records, look at the days you experienced flare-ups and compare them to days without flare-ups. See if there is one thing that always shows up on flare-up days and never appears on days without flare-ups. That, of course, is the simplest situation to deal with. Life is seldom simple, though.

It is important to only make one change at a time.

It is more likely you will find more than one different activity or food. Then you get to play amateur scientist. Pick one possible trigger—and only one—to eliminate. Keep records for a couple weeks to see if eliminating that one food or activity makes a difference.

If the pattern of flare-ups doesn't change at all, you can probably forget that as a possible trigger. If the pattern changes even a little, continue life without that possible trigger and choose one other possible trigger to eliminate.

It is important to make one change at a time, or you won't know what makes the difference. For example, if you start getting more sleep (which will likely reduce stress) and stop eating strawberries for breakfast in the same week, you can't tell if stress or strawberries were causing flare-ups.

After you have a good set of records, if your rosacea is so bad that you don't have many days without flare-ups, your baseline will be the days with flare-ups rather than good days. You will need to pick one thing to eliminate to see if that helps.

Check the list of common triggers to see if the most common are part of your daily life. You might as well start with the obvious! For instance, be religious about applying sun screen and wearing hats for a couple weeks to see if that helps decrease flare-ups. If the first thing you try doesn't seem to make a difference, work your way down the list—one item at a time. I think changing one thing for a week would be a good plan.

If your skin looks any better after a week, I'd give it another week or so before eliminating something else. See if the skin continues to improve.

Filling in the diary checklist should only take a couple minutes each night. Make it part of your routine at the end of the day.

I suggest getting an original from the National Rosacea Society by writing to National Rosacea Society, 800 S. Northwest Highway Suite 200, Barrington, IL 60010. You can reach them by phone at 847/382-8971. If you have access to the Internet, their Web page is at http://www.rosacea.org, where you can print a copy of the diary checklist. You can then make copies at the local quick print shop. Ask the quick print shop to punch holes in the copies and put the sheets in a three-ring binder.

If you have a pet theory about what might be causing your flare-ups, add that item on the back of the sheet and keep track of it, too. I've tried to give you enough information that if you discover a trigger not covered in the book, you might be able to figure out what is happening and how to minimize its effect.

Then keep the binder next to your bed, in the bathroom or anywhere convenient to bedtime routines. The investment of time and energy might make all the difference. Try to think of it as something you can do to take control of your condition and improve your life, instead of an imposed chore. No one is going to come around to see if you are keeping your diary checklist, but your bathroom mirror may tell you when you are doing a good job of it.

STRESS

Last, but certainly not least, is stress. Sixty percent of survey respondents said emotional stress triggered rosacea flare-ups. It was second only to the sun as the most common trigger—exposure to the sun scored 61%.

Emotional stress has two components: what happens to you, and how you choose to react to it. You can make choices that will affect how you react to stress.

Reducing stress in today's world may seem like an insurmountable task. Lots of people are working at it these days. The chapter on stress explains what happens to your body when you are under stress and provides some suggestions for coping with and reducing it. The stress chapter offers a basic sampler of approaches. If you see something that appeals to you, you may want to check out other books with more detail on the specific technique.

While medical treatment is important to living with rosacea, how you manage your life can be just as vital. Taking control of how you live will have rewards beyond keeping your skin and blood vessels healthy. This is particularly true when it comes to stress. I've never met anyone who said, "Gee, I wish I had more stress in my life."

It may turn out that rosacea is nature's way of telling you to slow down and enjoy yourself. Either relish the great life you have or build a great life you can enjoy.

EMOTIONAL IMPACT OF ROSACEA

A survey by the National Rosacea Society found as many as 75 percent of rosacea sufferers experienced loss of self-confidence after developing rosacea. Probably everyone with rosacea suffers some emotional effects of the condition. They can range from irritation to embarrassment to fear. Since rosacea tends to appear years after we thought we were done worrying about skin outbreaks, it is a pain in the neck to think about how what we eat may affect our skin. If your skin is very red, people may notice—even if they don't comment. Or, you may think everyone notices your permanent blush.

If you are one of those who develops rosacea in your forties or fifties, when you are struggling to cope with wrinkles—the rude reminders of time passing—the last thing you need is telangiectasia or a lumpy nose. One of my first reactions was, "Great! Another way my body is betraying me."

There is always the fear that anything out of the ordinary may be a sign of deeper trouble, too. There is no evidence that rosacea is a precursor of any serious illness. (You do want to check with your ophthalmologist to keep any ocular rosacea from damaging your eyes.) Even the most severe cases of rosacea skin involvement don't seem to lead to anything else.

As many as 75 percent of rosacea sufferers experienced loss of self-confidence after developing rosacea.

Even though you need to pay attention to activities and foods that cause flare ups, rosacea shouldn't change your life. You can do most of the things you have always done. That includes facing the world. Most people overestimate how much attention other people pay to them. A friend told me once not to worry so much about what other people thought of what I did. "They are too wrapped up in themselves to notice that much about you," she said.

If people do notice when you experience a flare up, you can do some public service work by explaining rosacea to them. While it seems to be more prevalent now, there are still lots of folks who haven't heard of it. Or have heard the name, but don't know exactly what it is.

Remember that stress is a prime trigger, so don't sit around stewing about rosacea. That isn't going to help. (Now I sound like my grandmother. Sorry.)

A PERSONAL STORY

I have no doubt that my rosacea is triggered by stress. As I approached my publisher's deadline for this book, my cheeks turned redder and tingled. The morning after I stayed up all night working on a particularly difficult section, a stye in my left eye popped out. When I was diagnosed with rosacea, I was working very hard on three big projects and having financial difficulties.

Just this morning, in the shower, I remembered my first chalazion. It was 25 years ago, long before I'd ever heard of rosacea. I don't remember any skin problems then, but ocular rosacea symptoms sometimes show up before the skin is involved. The doctor I saw cut out the chalazion and didn't say anything about its being a symptom of anything.

The interesting thing is to look back at my life at that moment in time. I was one year into a second marriage. We were having problems. We had just moved 2,000 miles across country. We were remodeling an old house we'd bought. My husband was working from 3 PM to midnight. I was going to school full-time, commuting an hour and a half each way. My three-year old daughter was not adjusting well to all the changes in her life.

I'm convinced that chalazion was not a coincidence. It was a signal no one understood.

CHAPTER 9
SKIN CARE

ROSACEA SUFFERERS SHOULD consider skin care to minimize flushing, protect the skin from weather and enhance general skin health. Healthy skin is more resistant to damage.

Skin is important for more than medical reasons. The appearance of the skin has social and psychological effects. We all want to look healthy and as attractive as possible. People react to our appearance.

Most of us have come to terms with not looking like a model, but we certainly don't want to look sickly or deformed. If rosacea is left untreated or mistreated, we risk permanent skin damage.

In addition to any advice from your dermatologist, here is some general information for minimizing skin damage from rosacea.

SKIN CARE ROUTINE

Whether you are used to scrubbing your face with a rough wash cloth lathered up with your bath soap, or using expensive, fragrant, lovely-colored cosmetics, you probably need to rethink your skin cleansing routine.

You don't want to rough up the skin while cleaning it. Because rosacea skin is fragile, the mechanics have to be gentle. Products are as important as the mechanics. As you'll see below, many common ingredients in skin care products tend to irritate rosacea skin.

Gentle actions with gentle products is the way to go. Resist the urge to clean your skin more frequently than twice a day. Rosacea is not a result of being unclean. Vigorous cleaning is apt to irritate your skin and the underlying tissues.

> *You probably need to rethink your skin cleansing routine.*

Here is a step-by-step routine for daily cleaning:

1. In the morning, wash your face with a mild cleansing agent. Avoid deodorant soaps and any product with alcohol. You may need to use a non-soap cleanser, if soap irritates your skin. Use warm, but not hot, water. Gently working the cleanser over your face with your fingertips is better than using a cloth or sponge. It is too easy to scrub hard with a cloth or sponge. Use plenty of water to make sure all the cleanser is rinsed off. Again, use warm water. Few of us end up with faces grimy enough to need a strenuous cleaning. Two gentle washings would be better than one vigorous one, if your face is

extremely dirty. Most of the time, one wash will be plenty.

2. Blot your face with a thick pile, cotton towel. Don't rub. Allow your face to air dry for several minutes before taking the next step.

3. Apply your topical medication with gentle strokes. There is no need to rub it deeply into the skin. Let that air dry for five to 10 minutes before you continue to the next step.

4. If you use moisturizer, apply it after the medication has thoroughly dried. Again, let it dry before you go on.

5. Sun screen is the next step. Daily sun screen use is recommended, even if you don't spend much time out of doors. After the sun screen is dry, apply makeup if you use it.

6. Your evening routine should include cleansing and medication as described in steps one and two above.

Adhering to a daily routine is your best chance of effectively controlling rosacea. Like any routine, it will become easier as time goes on if you stick with it.

Men might want to change to an electric shaver. Some find razor blades irritating. If you choose to stay with a blade, make sure you never use a dull one. Watch for irritation if you use the fancy blade razors that have aloe or other products applied to the blade. Avoid shaving lotions and creams that sting or burn.

BATHING AND SHOWERING

No more scalding baths or bracing cold showers for rosacea sufferers. Remember that
extremes in temperature can bring on flushing.
Some bath salts, bubble baths or bath herbs may
irritate your face. It might be better if you wait
to wash your face at the bathroom sink. Just pay
attention to see if your face gets red, tight or
itchy when you use bath products.

THE SUN AND ROSACEA

"The significance of sun-damaged skin in rosacea cannot be stressed enough," says a noted
German rosacea researcher.

A National Rosacea Society survey reported
sun exposure as a flare-up trigger for 61 percent of rosacea sufferers—the most widely
reported trigger. Sun exposure may damage
blood vessels as well as triggering flare-ups.

The sun's rays are hottest, most direct and
most damaging between 10 AM and 2 PM. Avoid
exposure to those rays. Sitting in the shade or
wearing a hat can help. Remember the sun's rays
are reflected by water, sand and snow. Those
reflected rays can damage the skin, too.

The best tactic for sun protection—after
avoidance—is wearing sun screen.

SUN SCREEN

Remember when everyone wanted the best tan?
Summer days were spent at the beach or lake,
working on a tan that would impress all our
friends. Most people understand now that is not
a good idea. The attractive brown skin is no
longer a sign of health, but rather an indication

of skin damage.

Rosacea sufferers should wear sun screen every day, not just when they head for the beach or ski slopes. Be sure to use a water-proof sun screen if you are going swimming.

Some sun screens include salicylic acid, which may be a flare-up trigger for rosacea sufferers. So read those labels, and watch for your personal reaction to products.

If regular sun screen irritates your skin, you could try one for young children. Another tactic that might help is to mix moisturizer with the sun screen.

Rosacea sufferers should wear sun screen every day.

An interesting point is much of the sun damage to our skin occurs before we are 18 years old. That makes sense because children are usually outside more than adults. When a lot of us were growing up, no one understood the dangers of sun exposure. Now that we do know, we should make sure children are protected when they are outdoors. The few moments invested in slathering on the sun screen today could provide them with the wealth of healthier skin as adults.

Use a sun screen with an SPF of at least 15. The SPF (sun protection factor) number tells you the level of sun protection from UVB rays (see below) it offers. An SPF of 15 means it will take 15 times as long to cause sun damage as going out unprotected.

Many sun screens offer protection only from ultraviolet B (UVB) rays. Ultraviolet A (UVA) rays also damage the skin. Look for a product that also offers UVA protection.

UVB AND UVA

UVB rays are the ones that cause sunburn. They also damage DNA and elastic tissues.

UVA rays accelerate the aging process. They cause premature wrinkling, age spots and photo aging, as well as damaging elastic tissues. UVA rays are present all year and can pass through glass, unlike UVB rays. They are longer than UVB rays and penetrate deeper into the skin.

Everyone should avoid both UVA and UVB ray exposure because they both cause elastic tissue damage. Elastic tissue damage is what gives some people that leathery, Marlboro Man look.

Rosacea sufferers probably should be most careful of UVA rays because they can penetrate deeper. Those delicate capillaries are already less elastic in rosacea sufferers and don't need exposure to any more threats.

Also notice that UVA rays can pass through glass, so sun screen is important even if you are stuck in an office or a truck all day long.

PABA

PABA (para-aminobenzoic acid) is commonly regarded as a skin irritant. Many suggestions for sensitive skin include avoiding products with PABA. While rosacea sufferers have sensitive skin, it isn't always your typical sensitive skin.

A study of sun screen/skin irritation among rosacea sufferers found that PABA wasn't the key ingredient to watch for. Researchers discovered it didn't seem to matter whether the sun screen had PABA or not.

The real difference between sun screens that didn't irritate rosacea sufferers' skin and those that did was whether the sun screen contained dimethicone and cyclomethicone or not. Products without dimethicone and cyclomethicone irritated the skin 14 times as much. So watch for dimethicone and cyclomethicone. You want a sun screen with these ingredients.

SKIN CARE PRODUCTS

Rosacea sufferers need to be careful with skin care products. A National Rosacea Society survey found 58 percent of people reported being sensitive skin care products. Another 24 percent reported being somewhat sensitive.

The frustrating thing is while rosacea sufferers need to use more products to protect their skin, there are more restrictions on which products they can safely use. It may take awhile and some testing to find out what is safe for you.

Good skin care for rosacea sufferers isn't about trying to look like a movie star or model. Even if you are a person who has taken pride in your lack of vanity, now is the time to pay some attention to your skin. If you don't, you risk facial deformity. I don't know anyone with so little vanity they wouldn't be bothered by that.

Generally rosacea sufferers should use skin care products that are water soluble, oil and fragrance free and nonabrasive. In general, it helps to choose facial products that won't clog pores: they will usually have the word "noncomedogenic" or "nonacneogenic" on the package. Many rosacea sufferers report being sensitive to common skin-care products, such as astringents, soaps, exfoliants, perfume, moisturizers, shaving cream, hair sprays and sun screen.

Back to the National Rosacea Society survey—here are the numbers on people bothered by various skin care products, sorted by gender:

WOMEN

49.5% reported sensitivity to astringents or toners

40% reported sensitivity to soap

34% reported sensitivity to exfoliant agents

29% reported sensitivity to makeup

27% reported sensitivity to perfume or cologne

25.5% reported sensitivity to moisturizer

20% reported sensitivity to hair spray

Skin Care Product Sensitivity--Women
National Rosacea Society survey

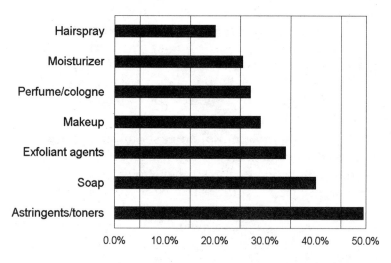

MEN

24% reported sensitivity to soap

19% reported sensitivity to perfume or cologne

13% reported sensitivity to sun screen

Skin Care Product Sensitivity--Men
National Rosacea Society survey

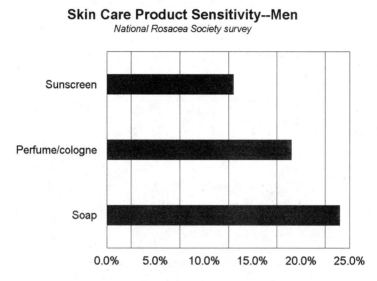

Twelve percent of men and women combined reported flare-ups caused by shampoo.

INGREDIENTS

Based on surveys done by the National Rosacea Society, here are some hints for skin care product ingredients to avoid. They were cited as skin irritants by people with rosacea. It is time to start reading labels carefully.

Topping the list as the most irritating ingredient by far was alcohol, as 66 percent of all respondents said alcohol burns, stings or aggravates their rosacea. Other commonly aggravating ingredients include witch hazel for 30 percent of the respondents, fragrance for 29.5 percent, menthol for 21 percent, peppermint for 14 percent and eucalyptus oil for 13 percent.

Despite the variety of skin-care products that may aggravate rosacea, the majority of respondents indicated they have been able to find the right products for their individual conditions.

Seventy-eight percent of the women said they are now using effective skin-care products that do not aggravate their rosacea, and 16 percent said this is sometimes the case. For men, the situation may be somewhat more challenging as 56 percent reported using suitable products and 21 percent said they are now using effective products that sometimes do not aggravate their rosacea.

You can do tests on your skin to see if they affect you. Even if they don't now, pay close attention to see if they begin to irritate your skin as rosacea progresses.

Skin Care Product Ingredient Irritants
National Rosacea Society survey

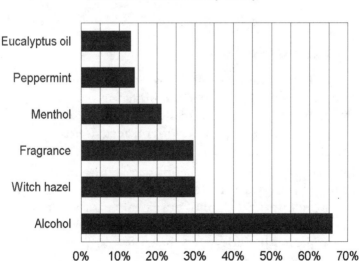

Potentially irritating ingredients to avoid include:

alcohol

clove oil

eucalyptus oil

menthol

peppermint

salicylic acid

witch hazel

Notice the natural ingredients like eucalyptus oil and peppermint on the list. Just because a product says it uses "all-natural" ingredients doesn't mean it will be good for you. You may come across recipes for homemade, "chemical-free" skin care products that are supposed to be safe for the "most sensitive" skin. If they contain any of the ingredients on the list, you may have a problem.

A lot of herbal remedies have salicylic acid, especially the oils and extracts. Be careful with the very popular natural cures for skin problems. Rosacea is more complicated than some other skin conditions because it involves the vascular system and underlying tissues.

Generally, any product that stings, burns or causes redness should be avoided.

ROSACEA-TARGETED PRODUCTS

I saw an ad for an all-natural soap while researching this book. The ad appeared in a glossy catalog of upscale products. The ad copy mentioned rosacea and implied the soap could cure rosacea.

The ad said "severe infestation [of *Demodex*] can cause a permanent, disfiguring condition known as Acne Rosacea." It quoted the *New York Times* with information about *Demodex*. It promised the soap would clear "your complexion without antibiotics." The ad included "before" and "after" pictures.

It was a pretty good ad.

The only problem is the soap probably won't cure your rosacea. Though *Demodex* has been implicated in rosacea, there is no solid evidence that it is the cause. [see Theories and Causes for more discussion of *Demodex*]

You are more apt to hear about the answer to rosacea on the news than to find it in a paid advertisement.

The ad doesn't list the ingredients of the herbal beauty soap, so I can't say it contains irritating substances—but that is a possibility. If the soap were available in a store, you could look at the label to check ingredients. Ordering a product like this without seeing what it contains would be a gamble.

Two bars of the soap cost $29.95! That is a hefty price for something that may not work.

As more people reach the age groups likely to develop rosacea, there are bound to be more products offered to the growing population of rosacea sufferers. The products will probably not be cheap. The sellers will have the money to pay for well-designed and well-written ads.

My recommendation is to think twice, or three times, before you spend your money on products that are hyped as cures or guaranteed treatments. If one product turns out to be the answer to rosacea, you are more apt to find about it on the news or in the paper than in a paid ad.

MAKEUP

If your rosacea affects your skin color enough to make you feel uncomfortable about your appearance, you should consider camouflage. The redness and telangiectasia can be hidden with a layer of green-tinted makeup under your regular makeup. You should be able to find the green-tinted prefoundation at a good cosmetic counter. It is usually available in either cream or liquid form. When you apply your regular foundation, any red tones should be hidden. I haven't tried this, but you might have to use a heavier skin-tone foundation than you normally use to completely cover the green-tint.

NOTE TO MEN

If your appearance is important to you, either for personal or professional reasons, you could consult a paramedical cosmetic consultant (an aesthetician) for suggestions about camouflage. I can hear some men muttering right now, "I don't need no stinking makeup." If you are in sales, for instance, and don't need any reason to feel less than absolutely confident in yourself and the impression you make, you should not feel uncomfortable about getting help for a medical condition. Just a suggestion.

COLD WEATHER SKIN CARE

Cold weather presents extra challenges to rosacea sufferers. Wind and cold temperatures tend to dry the skin more than warmer, moist air. You will find extra moisturizer might help protect the skin from winter cold.

When you go out, wrapping a scarf or muffler over the lower half of your face will shield your skin from the wind. If the weather is particularly bitter, or your skin is very sensitive, you may want to wear a ski mask (just be careful when you enter a bank!).

Moving from cold outside air to warmer inside air can cause flushing, too. As much as possible, you should make the change gradual. Loitering in your apartment lobby to look through your mail might help, since the lobby is probably cooler than your apartment. Spending a few moments close to the door when you enter any heated building will make the transition from cold to warm air less traumatic to your skin. It gives the body time to adjust to the change.

HOT WEATHER SKIN CARE

Hot weather can be as damaging to rosacea skin as cold weather. Sunlight tends to be brighter during hot weather, and sun is a major trigger of rosacea flare-ups. High temperatures cause flushing, especially during exertion.

In addition to protecting your skin from direct sun exposure with sun screen, a hat or other protective clothing, rosacea sufferers should drink extra fluids to make sure the body temperature doesn't rise. Chewing on ice chips can help keep you from becoming overheated.

When possible, you should spend time in air-conditioned places on hot, humid days. If you control the temperature settings, don't set them too cold. The change from air conditioning to the hot outside air can cause the same flushing as coming inside during cold weather.

Avoid heavy exercise during hot weather, especially if you exercise outdoors. It is better to exercise in the early morning or evening than during the middle of the day, when the sun is hottest and the temperatures highest. If you exercise inside, make sure the room is well ventilated and as cool as possible. When possible, run a fan or air conditioning. Draping a cold, damp towel around your neck can help you avoid being overheated. Spritzing your face with water from a spray bottle also helps.

If swimming is one of your hot weather activities, use waterproof sun screen. Be sure to rinse your face well when you leave the pool or ocean. Some rosacea sufferers have found chlorine and salt water irritating. Remember to reapply sun screen after rinsing.

CHAPTER 10
FOOD TRIGGERS

ROSACEA SUFFERERS HAVE found some foods act as triggers for flare-ups. Surveys re veal spicy and hot foods and beverages are common culprits. Other foods also trigger flare-ups—maybe because of ingredients or nutrients the rosacea sufferer's body has decided it just doesn't like. Foods you have eaten all your life may suddenly start bothering you.

A National Rosacea Society survey records the most common food triggers among respondents.

You may want to discover which foods are your triggers. Everyone does not react the same way. This seems particularly true with rosacea.

The rosacea diary checklist will come in handy for tracking what you have eaten before you experience a flare-up. Some people react within hours, but others may take longer. You might find there are cumulative effects, too. Maybe you can eat a little cheese, once in awhile, but if you eat cheese every day your skin will protest. The section on the diary checklist will give you details how to use this tool to track what bothers you.

There are some theories about why certain foods are more apt to cause rosacea flare-ups than others, but no clear cut answers yet. Alcoholic drinks can cause flushing in anyone, whether a rosacea sufferer or not. Hot drinks can raise body temperature, which causes flushing. Spicy foods can make you sweat and cause flushing. Foods with large amounts of naturally-occurring histamine can dilate the capillaries, which leads to flushing. Foods with high concentrations of niacin (vitamin B_3) can also cause flushing in some people.

Flare-up Trigger Foods
National Rosacea Society survey

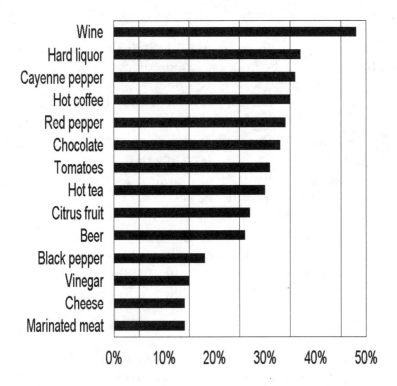

POSSIBLE TRIGGERS

Here is a longer list of foods that have triggered flare-ups in rosacea sufferers. There are a few extra ones that didn't make the National Rosacea Survey hit list.

avocados

bananas

cheese

citrus fruit

chocolate

eggplant

figs

lima beans

liver

navy beans

peas

raisins

red plums

spinach

sour cream

soy sauce

tomatoes

vanilla extract

vinegars

Some of the foods on the common trigger list share ingredients, and that might be clue about what is happening to your body when you eat them. It doesn't explain why the foods bother you, unfortunately. You'll just have to accept the fact that they do and get on with your life.

SALICYLIC ACID

Plums, raisins, tomatoes and vinegar appear on the common trigger list. They all contain salicylate. It is the salt form of salicylic acid, a natural chemical found in plants. They manufacture it to protect themselves from bacteria in the soil. Aspirin contains salicylic acid.

Salicylic acid is a great pain reliever. It brings down fever. It has been shown to help prevent heart disease. It may also be the reason some foods bring on a rosacea flare-up.

If plums, raisins, tomatoes or vinegar trigger flare-ups for you, take a look at the list below of other foods that may also bother you.

Careful monitoring of what you eat, and using the daily checklist, will help you identify your triggers. If several of the foods trigger a flare-up, you should probably watch for salicylic acid as an ingredient in cosmetics, hair care products and skin products.

Because the amount and strength of salicylic acid in various foods and products can vary so much, you may not have to avoid all of them. Just be aware of possible triggers.

Here are foods that contain salicylate in amounts that might trigger flare-ups:

almonds
apples
apple cider
apricots
blackberries
boysenberries
cherries
cloves

cucumbers

currants

gooseberries

grapes

green peppers

nectarines

oil of wintergreen

oranges

peaches

pickles

plums

prunes

raisins

raspberries

strawberries

tomatoes

tea

vinegar

Yellow food dye 5 (tartrazine) is similar to salicylic acid, but less potent. It is used to color cheese-flavored products, artificial fruit drinks and coatings on pills and candies.

Some prepared foods may use salicylates to add flavor, too. These include

bakery goods (other than bread)

cake mixes

candy

chewing gum

ice cream

jams

soft drinks

NIACIN

A couple of foods on the common trigger list are significant sources of niacin—avocados and liver. While niacin is a nutrient the body needs for normal growth, it appears to bother some rosacea sufferers. For this reason, there is a chance that other foods with high amounts of niacin may also act as flare-up triggers.

Interestingly, a reaction to an excess of niacin from supplements is facial flushing and skin tingling.

Foods high in niacin are lean meats, poultry, seafood, eggs, beans, and fortified breads and cereals. If these foods trigger a rosacea flare-up, taking an aspirin before eating should counteract the effect of niacin. Of course, if the salicylate in aspirin causes a flare-up, you are better off avoiding the niacin-rich foods. If you find you have to avoid them all together, taking a multi-vitamin is probably a good idea. Maybe the vitamin itself, removed from food, won't bother you.

HISTAMINE

The body reacts to histamine by dilating blood capillaries (which makes the skin redder) and making the capillaries more permeable, allowing fluid to escape into the underlying tissues. This fluid can cause swelling, damage the underlying tissue, and cause itchiness. Sound familiar? These match some of the mechanics of rosacea.

Histamine is generally linked to allergic reactions. People allergic to strawberries can break out in hives because of histamine. Mosquito bites itch because of histamine. On rare occasions, histamine can lead to anaphylaxis, an extreme reaction that can be fatal. There is no evidence that rosacea can cause anaphylaxis! I only mention it to show how powerful histamine can be.

In addition to foods that naturally contain histamine, the body also produces and releases histamine in reaction to what it sees as invaders. Pollen can trigger histamine release in some people.

Rosacea isn't generally considered an allergic condition, but the connection between histamine and food flare-up triggers is interesting. Some foods affect one rosacea sufferer, but not another—just like an allergy.

When the body releases histamine, it also prompts the stomach to produce more gastric acids. A study on *Helicobacter pylori* found rosacea sufferers suffer from more indigestion and consume more antacids than the general public does.

Foods containing histamine include:

- alcoholic beverages like beer, wines, vermouth
- avocados
- bananas
- processed beef
- cheeses
- chicken liver
- chocolate
- citrus fruits
- cider
- eggplant

figs

canned fish like anchovies, herring, mackerel, sardines and tuna

processed pork

raisins

sour cream

spinach

tomatoes

vinegar

yogurt

Some Oriental foods are also listed as those with histamine, but you will have to do some experimentation find out which ones affect you.

If the foods high in histamine appear to trigger rosacea flare-ups, taking an antihistamine an hour or so before eating them may lessen their effects.

Licorice (Glycyrrhiza glabra) is said to be a natural antihistamine. It not only reduces histamine release, it also inhibits its production. I don't think Good 'n Plenty is going to help, but one to two grams of powdered root three times a day might. Unfortunately, licorice is high in salicylates, too. Life will be easier for you if histamine and salicylates don't both bother you. If they do, I would stick with antihistamine pills rather than trying to make a "natural" ingredient work for you.

HOT AND SPICY FOODS

No matter what their ingredients, hot and spicy foods in general seem likely to bother rosacea sufferers. *Hot* in this case means hot in taste, not temperature. Some spices and peppers can make people actually break out in a sweat, so the mechanism of what is going on under the skin can be the same as what happens to rosacea sufferers during hot weather.

Hot and spicy foods seem likely to bother rosacea sufferers.

Even spices that don't make you sweat seem to trigger flare-ups in some people. Since a lot of spicy foods are Italian and Mexican with tomato bases, it might be the tomatoes that are actually bothering you. If you want to minimize the foods you need to eliminate from your diet, it may take some clever detective work to pinpoint exactly what is triggering the flare-ups.

The National Rosacea Society suggests some substitutes for spices that might cause flare-ups. If curry powder bothers you try concocting a substitute made of 2 teaspoons of cumin combined with 1 teaspoon of oregano.

For poultry seasoning you could substitute a mixture of ½ teaspoon sage, ½ teaspoon coriander, ¼ teaspoon thyme, ½ teaspoon basil or oregano, and ½ teaspoon marjoram.

Make your own curry powder substitute of 4 teaspoons coriander, 2 teaspoons turmeric, 1 teaspoon cinnamon, 1 teaspoon cumin, ½ teaspoon basil or oregano, and ½ teaspoon cardamom.

BEVERAGES

Alcoholic beverages are frequent rosacea flare-up triggers. Wine affected almost half of the rosacea sufferers who responded to the National Rosacea Society survey. Since the wines most people drink are made from grapes, it makes sense that wine and raisins are both triggers. Grapes contain salicylate. Alcohol also dilates blood vessels. Red wine seems to bother more people than white.

Hard liquor like bourbon, gin and vodka also tend to trigger flare-ups. Beer can, also. The National Rosacea Society survey didn't mention whether it takes more beer to trigger a flare-up than hard liquor. Since beer contains less alcohol, ounce for ounce, than hard liquor it would be interesting to see if you can drink more beer without triggering.

Hot non-alcoholic drinks also trigger flare-ups in more than a third of survey respondents. The temperature of the drinks seems to be the trigger factor. Hot coffee and tea can bother rosacea sufferers. If you drink them slightly cooler, that may be the only change you need to make. At least one study concluded it wasn't the caffeine in coffee and tea that bothered rosacea sufferers.

Hot chocolate may be a different story, because chocolate at any temperature may be a trigger. If you love your hot chocolate, maybe serving it cooler with less chocolate will work.

MARINATED MEATS

The alcohol in marinated meats may be the reason they bother some rosacea sufferers. Some alternatives would be to use mild spices to flavor meat instead of marinades. If you grill meat, try adding mesquite or smoked wood chips to the charcoal instead.

GENERAL FOOD FLUSHING

No matter what the specific foods are, eating a heavy meal can cause flushing. The demands of digesting a lot of food at once create stress and excess blood flow to the face. Eating smaller meals throughout the day would be better than eating an enormous dinner.

Eating a lot of sugar at once can have the same effect as alcohol (well, maybe not exactly the same!) on the blood vessels. Because these simple carbohydrates enter the blood stream quickly, they cause glucose spikes which dilate the blood vessels. Eating high fiber foods with foods high in sugar helps delay digestion and cuts back on the amount of glucose rushing into the blood system.

Sugar comes in various forms. Many of them have names that end in -ose: sucrose, lactose, maltose, fructose, glucose and dextrose. Ingredients on labels that include the word syrup are usually a form of sugar, too. Molasses and honey also fall into the sugar category.

TIPS FOR DINING OUT

Dining out can be especially challenging for many rosacea sufferers. But by paying attention to your selection of foods and beverages, you may be able to avoid ordering a rosacea flare-up. Here are some tips to make your meal more pleasurable without bringing home a rosacea doggy bag:

Choose restaurants that offer rosacea-friendly menus. Many rosacea sufferers must avoid hot spicy foods such as those made with white and black pepper, paprika, red pepper and cayenne. So, in general, avoid restaurants that specialize in that type of cuisine.

Select your meal based on your own personal knowledge of items that may cause a flare-up in your case. Although those chips and salsa may taste great, if hot spices aggravate your condition, are they worth the ravages of rosacea? Some foods, such as tomatoes, spinach or chocolate, contain histamine or agents that cause the release of histamine in the body, which may trigger a flare-up in some sufferers. Foods containing niacin, such as liver, also may cause flushing in some individuals.

If you're not sure how an item is prepared, ask your server to help you avoid ingredients that may affect you.

Eliminate or minimize alcoholic beverages if they aggravate your condition.

Avoid thermally hot beverages. Selecting cold drinks, or allowing hot coffee or tea to cool, may help avoid a flare-up.

Remember, although the list of possible rosacea triggers is long, what may cause a flare-up in one person may have no effect on another.

Why do some foods prompt rosacea? Anything consumed that brings on flushing—most commonly spicy foods or thermally hot beverages—can be a culprit in inducing a flare-up. And a vast array of other foods, while less common as trip wires, has also been found to affect various individuals.

Foods containing histamine or those that release histamine in the body—such as tomatoes, spinach, eggplant, cheese, chocolate, chicken livers, citrus fruits, bananas, raisins, figs, avocados, yogurt and sour cream—or foods containing niacin, can cause flushing. Foods high in niacin include liver and yeast.

Here are some tips when selecting your meal:

"Hot" spices such as white and black pepper, paprika, red pepper and cayenne are common rosacea trip wires. Look for substitutes. Marinated meat, vanilla, soy sauce, vinegar, red plums, and the pods of broad-leaf beans, such as limas, navy or peas, have been found to affect some rosacea sufferers. Taking an antihistamine about two hours before a meal that includes a food high in histamine, or an aspirin before eating a niacin-containing food may be helpful.

It is the heat in beverages, rather than other substances such as caffeine, that may directly bring on a flare-up. So reducing the temperature may be all that's necessary.

CHAPTER 11
NUTRITION

THOUGH THERE IS NO EVIDENCE that nutrition plays an active role in rosacea, it only makes sense to eat right so your skin and blood vessels are as healthy as possible. If they are in the best shape, maybe they will be able to resist the ravages of rosacea.

Some of the foods listed below may be flare-up triggers for you. You will have to observe your reaction to see if each is good for you. If a particular food does cause a flare-up, try introducing another nutrient source from the same group and see what happens.

Many people believe it is better to get nutrients from whole foods, rather than supplements, but if the food causes a flare-up you might have to use supplements to get the nutrient.

VITAMIN A

Your body makes vitamin A from beta carotene and retinols. Beta carotene comes from plant foods; retinols come from animal products. Vitamin A is important to the skin as well as the gums, glands, bones and teeth. Body cells need vitamin A to develop properly. The recommended daily allowance is 1 mg for men and 800 mcg (or .8 mg) for women. Signs of deficiency connected to rosacea are dry skin and eyes. The body stores vitamin A in the liver and fatty tissue for as long as three months, so it is possible to overdose on it. It probably isn't a good idea to take extra vitamin A without consulting your medical practitioner. Symptoms of excess vitamin A are headaches and blurred vision, bone and joint pain, appetite loss, diarrhea, rashes, itchiness, cracked skin, and hair loss. Women of childbearing age need to be especially careful, because excess vitamin A just before or in the early months of pregnancy can cause birth defects.

Good sources of vitamin A are:

apricots

asparagus

beans

cantaloupe

carrots

cheddar cheese

citrus fruits

egg yolks

leafy green vegetables

organ meats

peas

pumpkin

squash

salmon

tuna

yogurt

VITAMIN C

Vitamin C is an antioxidant, which some believe reduces cell destruction from oxidation. It helps build collagen, the supportive tissue under the skin. It strengthens blood vessel walls, including capillaries. It is also supposed to provide some anti-histamine action. (I find it confusing that some of the foods high in vitamin C are also on the list of foods that have histamine in them! I'm guessing it is another one of life's little mysteries.) Since histamines are suspected of being involved in capillary damage, vitamin C is very important for capillary health.

Good sources of vitamin C are:

broccoli

cabbage

cantaloupe

citrus fruit

green leafy vegetables

kiwi fruit

peas

peppers

potatoes

strawberries

sweet potatoes

tomatoes

yams

VITAMIN E

This is another antioxidant—according to one study, it is three times better than vitamin C. It is also necessary for calcium absorption, which promotes strong teeth and bones. Women who take estrogen after menopause may suffer from vitamin E deficiencies. The daily recommended allowance is 10 mg for men and 8 mg for women. Excessive bleeding is a symptom of excess vitamin E.

Good sources for vitamin E are:

almonds

avocados

fortified cereals

eggs

green leafy vegetables

lima beans

margarine

mayonnaise

nuts

oat bran

peaches

peanut butter

rice bran

salmon

shrimp

soybeans

sunflower seeds

wheat bran

wheat germ

COPPER

Copper is good for the skin and is a natural antihistamine. It is essential for healthy red blood cells, connective tissue, nerve fibers and skin pigmentation. Too little copper makes blood vessels inelastic. This makes it a nutrient rosacea sufferers should probably pay attention to. Daily recommended allowances haven't been established, but the National Academy of Sciences suggests 1.5 mg to 3 mg for both men and women. Anemia is a symptom of deficiency. Vomiting, diarrhea and liver disease are symptoms of excess copper.

Good sources of copper are:

legumes

liver

molasses

nuts

prunes

shellfish

soybeans

NIACIN (B$_3$)

This B vitamin is important for the metabolism and the production of DNA, protein and fatty acids. Additionally, niacin may inhibit histamine production. That could be a plus if you are sensitive to histamine. The recommended daily allowance is 19 mg for men and 15 mg for women.

There are no easy recommendations about niacin. Some rosacea sufferers seem to be sensitive to niacin and have flare-ups after eating food high in niacin. If niacin doesn't bother you, but foods with histamine seem to, it is probably a good idea to eat foods with niacin at the same meals you eat the foods with histamine.

Good sources of niacin are:

poultry

seafood

nuts

fortified cereals and breads

OMEGA-3 FATTY ACIDS

Omega-3 fatty acids help to reduce skin inflammation and help with eye health. They also allow cell membranes to transport nutrients in and out of cells. High doses of Omega-3 fatty acids can inhibit blood platelet function and decrease blood clotting. If you start bruising easily and have increased your intake of Omega-3 fatty acids, you might want to cut back again. A blood test can determine if your platelet count is low.

Good sources of Omega-3 fatty acids are:

canola oil

collards

eggs

flax oil and seeds

kale

mustard greens

nuts

pumpkin seeds

salmon

soybeans

spinach

tuna

wheat germ

Evening primrose oil is a good source of Omega-3 fatty acids, too. Fish oil supplements might not be a good idea, because they can inhibit clotting that, in turn, can lead to bleeding problems. Since rosacea sufferers' capillaries are already fragile, it would be best to avoid fish oil supplements. If you want to try evening prim-rose oil, pay close attention to your reaction to it. Herbal oils tend to trigger rosacea flare-ups in some people.

An extra benefit of Omega-3 fatty acids is they stimulate the metabolism and speed up the burn-ing of fats and glucose. That might help you lose some extra weight.

FLAX SEEDS AND OIL

Flax promotes healthy skin. You can get the ben-efits from a daily tablespoon of flax oil or two tablespoons of flax seed meal. The oil may be easier to deal with than grinding flax seeds, but the oil tends to go rancid within six weeks. An-other reason to go for the seeds is that flaxseed oil may contain more salicylic acid—a flare-up trigger for some rosacea sufferers.

If you buy oil, buy only small light-proof con-tainers and store them in the refrigerator. Flax oil can be added to smoothies (blended whole fruit or vegetable drinks) or taken by the spoon-ful. It boosts the power of food rich in amino acids if taken with them. Yogurt, cabbages, meat, seafood and soy products are enhanced by add-ing flax oil.

Flax seeds contain additional nutrients that don't survive the oil extraction. If you take the time to grind flax seeds in a coffee grinder and sprinkle the meal on salads or cereal, you will be doing your skin a big favor.

RIBOFLAVIN

One of the vitamin Bs, riboflavin contributes to healthy skin and aids in relieving stress (a com-mon emotional rosacea trigger). Some people have reported a lessening of rosacea symptoms after taking large doses of riboflavin.

Good sources of riboflavin are:

almonds

artichokes

beet greens

broccoli

fortified cereals and breads

cheese

fish

green leafy vegetables

meat

milk

potatoes

poultry

spinach

sweet potatoes

tofu

wheat germ

yogurt

SELENIUM

This antioxidant works with vitamin E to protect cell membranes. It is also said to boost the body's immune system. Since some rosacea researchers have described rosacea as possibly an autoimmune disease, it might be a good idea to take a supplement of chelated selenium, or at least a multivitamin with selenium. It is also supposed to encourage tissue elasticity. (Maybe it will help those poor capillaries.) One source suggest 200 micrograms (mcg) a day, but the recommended daily allowance is only 70 mcg for men and 55 mcg for women. Signs of excess selenium include diarrhea, nausea, abdominal pain, tooth damage, fatigue, irritability, and hair and nail loss.

Good sources of selenium are:

brazil nuts

brewer's yeast

chicken white meat

cottage cheese

egg yolks

garlic

lamb chops

lobster

nuts

onions

red snapper

shrimp

sunflower seeds

tuna

wheat germ

WATER

One of the basic elements the body needs but which is often overlooked is water. It has no nutrients or calories, but virtually all body functions use water. Blood plasma (the watery component of blood) uses about three liters of water to transport nutrients to all the cells. The average body needs about 30 liters of water to circulate within all the cells in the body. Another twelve liters of water circulates around the cells.

Water helps digestion and elimination, lubricates organs and joints, provides a protective cushion around cells, and helps keep the skin soft and pliable. It also helps regulate body temperature. That can reduce your risk of becoming overheated—a common rosacea flare-up trigger.

Be sure you drink six to eight 8-ounce glasses of water each day.

ZINC

This mineral helps the skin regenerate. It has been praised as an aphrodisiac, too, so maybe you will get a bonus from making sure you and your loved one get enough zinc. Bran and some whole-grain products and legumes contain phytates that inhibit the body's absorption of zinc. The daily recommended allowance is 15 mg for men and 12 mg for women. Among people who eat moderately balanced diets, deficiency is rare. Too much may actually inhibit the immune system. An excess can also cause nausea, vomiting, heart muscle damage and kidney failure.

Good sources of zinc are:

beef

crab

dark poultry meat

fish

fortified cereals

organ meats

oysters

pumpkin seeds

squash seeds

wheat germ

yogurt

CHAPTER 12
STRESS

ONE OF THE MORE FREQUENTLY mentioned rosacea flare-up triggers is stress. It is second only to sun exposure—and a very close second. Sixty percent of people who participated in a National Rosacea Society survey cited emotional stress as a trigger.

We all have heard how much stress affects our lives. In addition to making us irritable and less productive, it can have profound effects on overall health. People are dying every day from stress-related illnesses. For years heart attack and stroke were known as possible consequences of too much stress. Now we are starting to learn how stress is involved in many other diseases. It shouldn't be surprising that rosacea is among them.

Learning how to reduce stress in your life will do more than relieve rosacea symptoms. It just may prolong your life. It will certainly make you easier to live with! You could start a ripple effect, too. As you become easier to live with, you might relieve some of the stress in other people's lives.

Stress is not all bad, of course. A little bit of stress gets you moving. It is only when the stress is overpowering or prolonged that it causes problems.

PROS AND CONS OF STRESS

Our bodies became programmed to respond to threats with stress thousands of years ago. When we left the cave to go hunting for berries or meat, we might have encountered a wild animal or human enemy. Threats like that called for drastic measures if we wanted to safely return to the cave we called home.

Under stress the heart beats faster to send more blood to the muscles for added strength. The thyroid goes into overdrive to speed up the metabolism for extra energy. The blood gets thicker so it can carry more oxygen to the muscles, and so bleeding from wounds will clot faster.

Those reactions to danger were useful when threats were animals with sharp teeth and folks with heavy clubs. They don't work so well against an impatient boss, heavy traffic or a whining child. In fact, they are pretty darn useless. Stress gets us ready for "fight or flight." In most cases, we can neither fight nor fly away from the stresses we experience.

Prolonged stress exhausts the body.

Not only are they useless, they can be harmful. The reactions to stress work well for immediate, temporary danger. They aren't so good for the body over a sustained time. When our bodies created the reactions, threats were temporary. The stresses most of us experience these days are not short term. Stress has become a way of life.

When the body remains under stress for prolonged periods, faster heart beats can lead to high blood pressure, faster metabolism can lead to physical exhaustion and insomnia, thicker blood can cause circulatory problems including blood clots leading to stroke. Prolonged stress also exhausts the body. It uses up our resources, leaving us mentally and physically drained.

Stress has been found to damage the immune system, leaving us more vulnerable to disease and less able to heal.

STRESS AND ROSACEA

Here's one way stress relates directly to rosacea. When the body is under stress, it produces adrenaline or epinephrine. A study found that epinephrine promotes the release of bradykinin by the body. [Still with me?] Bradykinin is a substance the body makes to increase vascular permeability and dilate blood vessels. Hence, the flush.

Some of us have an Uncle Frank who gets all red in the face when he discusses politics or the general decline of Western civilization. Others of us suffer from rosacea and get red faces from less dramatic causes.

Stress is not good for you. I suppose we could look at rosacea as an early warning system. Some people don't realize they have too much stress in their lives until they have a heart attack. It seems likely we would get the message in the mirror.

RATING YOUR STRESS

Aside from the frustrations of life that you probably recognize as causing stress, changes in your life also contribute to stress. Even good things. The following table was created by two American doctors, T.H. Holmes and R.H. Rahe, to evaluate how much stress you have in your life.

The table lists events and assigns a stress score to each event. The scores are based on studies of many people, so they will vary from person to person. It is probably most helpful just to see how different events stack up relative to each other. You may not have considered some event as stressful.

If you want to score yourself, check off how many of the events have happened to you in the past year. A score of 300 or higher is supposed to put you at high risk of developing a health problem. A score of 150 or lower should indicate a manageable amount of stress in your life.

THE HOLMES-RAHE SCALE

LIFE EVENT	SCORE
Death of spouse	100
Divorce	75
Marital separation	65
Imprisonment	63
Death of a close family member	63
Personal injury or illness	53
Marriage	50
Dismissal from work	47
Marital reconciliation	45
Retirement	45
Change in health of family member	44

Pregnancy	40
Sexual difficulties	39
Gain of new family member	39
Business readjustment	39
Change in financial state	38
Change in frequency of arguments with spouse	35
Major mortgage	32
Foreclosure of mortgage or loan	30
Change in responsibilities at work	29
Son or daughter leaving home	29
Trouble with in-laws	29
Outstanding personal achievement	28
Spouse begins or stops work	26
Begin or end school	26
Change in living conditions	25
Revision of personal habits	24
Trouble with boss	23
Change in working hours or conditions	20
Change in residence	20
Change in schools	20
Change in recreation	19
Change in church activities	19
Change in social activities	18
Minor mortgage or loan	17
Change in sleeping habits	16
Change in number of family reunions	15
Change in eating habits	15
Vacation	13
Christmas	12
Minor violation of the law	11

DEALING WITH STRESS

There are a dozen, if not more, ways to deal with stress. The best may be to remove the source of stress. That isn't always practical, but might be worth examining as a possibility. If your job is always stressful, you may be in the wrong job or working for the wrong person. If your marriage is stressful more often than not, you and your spouse should probably try to figure out what is wrong.

One approach to eliminating stress is to simplify your life. Cut back on your obligations. Downscale your career or financial goals. Don't try to be a superman or superwoman by satisfying everyone else's needs at the expense of your own.

Stress is not so much what happens to you, but how you react.

Eliminating sources of stress is a big issue. Only you can decide what is appropriate for you. Dealing with stress has techniques you can learn and practice without major changes in your life. You may find changes follow after you aren't so stressed, though. They are more likely to be positive changes than not.

Since you probably won't be able to eliminate all the sources of stress in your life, you'll have to find new ways of dealing with it. What causes stress is not so much what happens to you, but how you react to what is happening to you.

The next time you are stuck in traffic, take a look at the drivers around you. Some will be scowling, with darting eyes searching for an open space in the next lane. Others will be calmly waiting to move on, maybe listening to the radio or talking to a passenger. The scowlers are not necessarily the more powerful people with more pressing deadlines to meet.

Reacting to stress with impatience doesn't mean you are a busy, powerful person. That is a lesson I'm still working on. Somewhere in the darkest recesses of my brain, being stressed means I have important things to do—so I must be important. The brighter side of my brain recognizes that feeling stressed just means I'm not maintaining control of my life.

A tricky aspect of stress is that it feeds on itself. If you feel pressured, anything that doesn't go just right adds to your stress. You need to break the cycle. Learning relaxation techniques and exercises can help you do that. Spending a few minutes a day clearing out residual stress puts you in better shape to deal with what life deals out.

Some people find doing the exercises in the morning gives them the resources they need to face the day. Others do the exercises in the evening to decompress after a day in the world. The super-stressed or over-achievers do them in the morning and evening. Maybe a few minutes at lunch would come in handy, too. Play with a schedule and see what benefits you.

After you get over the shock of not being stressed, you might find the relaxation exercises just feel so good you want to do them several times a day, as your schedule permits.

RELAXATION EXERCISES

Some of these are more elaborate than others. For some you'll want to find a quiet place where you can be alone and undisturbed. Others can be done in just a few moments at your desk.

MEDITATION VACATION

Sit in a dimly-lit room in a comfortable chair.

Close your eyes and let your thoughts wander. Relax and let go (this gets easier with practice, trust me).

After a minute, open and then close your eyes. Breathe deeply and slowly. Continue to let your mind drift.

After another minute, open your eyes for about 30 seconds. Then close them again. Keep breathing deeply and slowly.

Now, concentrate on a pleasant thought. Anything that is pleasant for you. There is no "right" thought (thinking of how nice it will be to be done with the nonsense of a meditation vacation might qualify as a not-right thought, but anything else goes). Imagine an image or sound that goes with that thought.

Concentrate on the image or sound until you feel yourself relaxing. If you focus on that one thing, it will be harder for other thoughts to intrude. With practice, this gets easier.

Continue concentrating for eight minutes. You can sneak a peek at the clock to check the time. Stressed people usually are amazed at how slowly those eight minutes pass. It may be hard to maintain your concentration for that long, but you can do it. And...with practice, it gets easier.

After eight minutes of focusing on the image or sound, slowly open your eyes, exhale deeply and slowly stand up.

You should feel invigorated. If you don't, that doesn't mean you are a bad person—it just means you need more practice. Congratulate yourself for actually finishing the exercise, and try again tomorrow.

SELF-HYPNOSIS

You don't have to go to a night club to be hypnotized. No one will tell you to cluck like a chicken every time you hear the word 'mother.' Hypnosis has outgrown its show business stage. Professional hypnotists are supposed to get pretty good results helping people quit smoking, lose weight and deal with other issues.

You can use self-hypnosis for relaxation. You won't go into a trance. You will still be aware of what is going on around you. You will be able to easily stop any time you want to. You'll find it is similar to the meditation vacation, but the mechanics are slightly different.

Sit in a comfortable chair, close your eyes and breathe deeply.

Focus on an object in front of you. Some people like to look at a crystal or flickering candle. It doesn't matter. If you want to focus on the TV or yesterday's newspaper, that is fine.

Breathe rhythmically, focus on your object, and tell yourself (silently) you feel relaxed and at peace. Feel your arms and legs become heavier as you relax.

When you are completely relaxed, drag out that pleasant thought from the meditation vacation or visualize a beautiful scene (maybe the lake where you spent summers when you were growing up, or a place you never been but have created in your mind). Let the thought or scene fill your mind. Again, concentrating on a pleasant thing forces out the bad stuff.

There is no set time for this exercise. Stay in your "pleasant place" for as long as you like. When you are ready to return to the real world, gradually expand your attention so you aren't focusing. Sit quietly for a moment before you re-enter the daily grind—now better equipped to cope with what faces you.

PROGRESSIVE RELAXATION

Here's simple relaxation exercise.

Sit down, close your eyes and do nothing for a minute or two.

Open your eyes for about 20 seconds, close them again and do nothing for another couple minutes.

Open your eyes for 10 to 30 seconds.

Close your eyes and concentrate on your scalp.

Inhale deeply through your nose and tense your scalp muscles.

Exhale through your nose and relax your

scalp muscles.

Keep moving down your body, relaxing muscles. Do your forehead next, then your cheeks.

Relax your neck, shoulders, upper back, lower back, arms, hands, fingers, diaphragm, abdomen, pelvis, thighs, lower legs, feet and finally your toes. You may need as long as 15 minutes to get from your scalp to your toes.

Take ten deep breaths and think of something pleasant for a few minutes before getting up.

YOGA

Developed in India more than 5,000 years ago, yoga is still going strong. It must have something going for it, eh? Whether you want to accept the philosophical side of yoga or not, the exercises can relieve stress with their slow, deliberate movements.

Breathing properly is very important in yoga. Serious practitioners believe the life energy (prana) flows through our bodies by our breathing. Breathe steadily and do the following exercise in continuous movements. There is no jerk and pull in yoga.

This yoga exercise is called the moon asana posture. If you have high blood pressure, you should NOT do this.

Kneel on the floor and sit on your heels.

Behind your back, grasp your right wrist with your left hand.

Inhale, and then, as you exhale, slowly

bend forward from your hips until your forehead touches the floor—or as close as you can get. (If you don't reach the floor the first time you try this, find something comfortable to place on the floor to rest your head on. After a while, your flexibility should get better, so you will be able to reach the floor.)

Let go of your wrist, allowing your arms to fall to the floor next to your legs.

Remain in that position for a moment or two.

Slowly inhale and lift yourself up until you are in an upright kneeling position.

If yoga appeals to you, there are many books and videos available to learn more postures.

EXERCISE

In general, a regular exercise routine is a good remedy for stress. Rosacea sufferers have to watch out for flushing, so you need to develop a routine that isn't too strenuous. Rosacea isn't an excuse to turn into a couch potato, though. There are many low-impact, non-aerobic exercise regimens that relieve stress and build good health.

SLEEP

Proper rest is important in stress management. If your body is tired, it doesn't deal with anything as well as it could. Sleep does more than rest the body, as well. While we sleep the body makes necessary repairs to cells. The brain needs the rest, too. Even when we don't feel sleepy, without adequate sleep we don't think as clearly and quickly.

Recent studies report that most Americans are sleep-deprived. As work- and family-related activities demand more time, sleep is a common casualty.

The theory is that if you are getting enough sleep, you don't need an alarm clock to wake up in the morning. (I guess I have spent my whole life sleep-deprived, if that is true!)

Studies report most Americans are sleep-deprived.

If getting to sleep is a problem for you, the sleep experts have some tips.

Go to bed at the same time each night.

Develop a bedtime routine that signals it is time to sleep (remember doing that when your kids were little? It works for adults, too).

Don't watch TV or do paperwork in bed.

Make sure the temperature of the bedroom is comfortable.

If you have a street light right outside the bedroom window, close the blinds or drapes.

There is conflicting advice about what to do if you wake up in the night and can't get back to sleep. One school of thought is to get up and do something quiet for a few minutes before going back to bed.

Another sleep researcher suggests you remain in bed, and resist the urge to look at the clock to see what time it is. She says if you keep your eyes closed, you have a better chance of going back to sleep soon.

We've all heard that as we age, we need less sleep. The newest research says that isn't true. Older people tend to wake up earlier because of changes in the internal clock, but they should still be getting seven to nine hours of sleep each night. That means going to bed earlier, if you are going to be waking up at the crack of dawn. (Another one of Mother Nature's cruel jokes, that retired people naturally wake up earlier after they don't have to be at the office by eight.)

RECREATION

Doing fun stuff is a stress reducer. If you don't have a hobby, find one. Doing something different from your job is actually more relaxing and rejuvenating than doing nothing. If your job is physical, try a sedentary activity like genealogy or stamp collecting. If you spend your work day sitting in front of a computer, take up gardening or something else that requires a little movement.

Get out of the house on your days off, instead of watching TV. A change of scenery and routine is a good way to break the stress cycle. Going to the movies, touring a museum or visiting friends will recharge your batteries.

CHAPTER 13
TREATMENT

DERMATOLOGISTS SEEM TO BE consistent in their treatment of rosacea—a regimen of both oral and topical antibiotics is pretty standard. The antibiotics generally prove to be successful in controlling the progress of rosacea.

In a study of 113 patients with papules, pustules, telangiectasia and moderate to severe facial erythema treated with oral tetracycline and metronidazole gel, 92% displayed fewer papules and pustules after treatment. Papules and pustules were totally eliminated in 59% of patients. Seventy-three percent of the patients ended up with less erythema.

Ongoing treatment is vital with rosacea. The medication alleviates symptoms effectively for the majority of rosacea sufferers who continue using it. It is important to remember that antibiotics don't cure rosacea, so you are never done taking them.

The disease goes in and out of remission, or periods of not exhibiting symptoms, but studies have found it never goes away. Rosacea sufferers who discontinue their medication may go for a time without symptoms, especially if they are very careful about avoiding flare-up triggers. Others who stop using the medicines exhibit symptoms within days.

You should discuss treatment with your dermatologist to determine how much of a bad idea it is for you to discontinue your medicine. You may have other medical conditions that complicate the situation, or your rosacea may be in the very early, mild stage. There could be dozens of reasons why it would be all right or even desirable for you to discontinue medication, but you need to talk to your doctor first.

ANTIBIOTICS

Several different antibiotics have been used to treat rosacea for years. They include tetracycline, clarithromycin, doxycycline, metronidazole and tretinoin. Some of these medications are available in both oral/systemic (taken by mouth, affecting the entire body) and topical (applied to the skin, mostly affecting only the area treated) forms.

It doesn't seem to be absolutely clear why antibiotics work so well for rosacea. Since a bacterial cause hasn't been established for rosacea, it doesn't quite make sense to us non-medical types that they are effective. One possible explanation is that the anti-inflammatory properties of antibiotics play the largest role in relieving symptoms.

Oral antibiotics appear to be effective in treating ocular rosacea.

Long-term use of oral antibiotics makes some

people nervous. Some people worry they will develop a tolerance to the medicine and will have to take increasingly larger doses. That doesn't seem to have happened with people taking antibiotics for rosacea.

Another concern about antibiotic use is bacteria's building up resistance to the medicine so it no longer is effective against them.

Side effects are yet another concern. While the antibiotics are killing bad stuff, they also can destroy helpful bacteria in the intestines, stomach and female genital area. Killing off the good guys upsets the delicate balance of internal organisms and can lead to diarrhea, digestive troubles and yeast infections.

There are indications that some antibiotics diminish birth control pills' power. There don't seem to be any studies to prove it, because researchers haven't found enough women willing to take birth control pills and antibiotics at the same time to see if they get pregnant. Doctors have noticed that birth control pills fail more often when women take certain antibiotics. Make sure you talk to your doctor about the interaction, if you are taking birth control pills.

Discuss any of your concerns with your doctor. In my research, I didn't find answers to them. It appears they are legitimate issues that have to be taken into consideration when determining a treatment plan that works for you.

Here is some information about the most commonly prescribed drugs for rosacea.

CLARITHROMYCIN

This seems to help rosacea sufferers because of its anti-inflammatory effects. Inflammation of capillaries and underlying skin tissue lead to erythema, telangiectasia and facial swelling. One study found clarithromycin caused fewer side effects than systemic tetracycline and metronidazole.

Clarithromycin also affects *Helicobacter pylori,* which has been found in a certain percentage of rosacea sufferers' gastric juices. Interestingly, the dosage that helps rosacea is much smaller than the one that eradicates *Helicobacter pylori.*

Clarithromycin provides dramatic results when prescribed for steroid rosacea.

A research study mentioned that the effectiveness of clarithromycin coupled with its lessened side effects "reward" the cost of treatment. Though scientists don't usually discuss such mundane matters as patients' expenses, I think it is fair to guess this drug must be expensive.

If you suffer side effects from the more commonly prescribed medications, you might discuss clarithromycin with your doctor.

DOXYCYCLINE

Some dermatologists report good success with doxycycline in treating rosacea. One reason for its success may be better patient compliance when it comes to taking the medication. Doxycycline doesn't have to be taken on an empty stomach, as some other antibiotics do. Taking doxycycline with milk cuts down on the possibility of stomach upset.

Some patients report increased sensitivity to the sun while taking doxycycline. Taking the medication at night, rather than in the morning, may help decrease the odds of experiencing the side effect.

TETRACYCLINE

Conventional treatment for rosacea has included tetracycline for three decades. It has been effective in many cases and may be the most commonly prescribed drug for rosacea. It has side effects, though. It may make the skin very sensitive to the sun. Pregnant and breast-feeding women should not take tetracycline.

Because tetracycline has been successfully used for so long, I couldn't find any current research on the drug.

METRONIDAZOLE

This antibiotic is available in both oral and topical forms. A common treatment plan includes oral tetracycline and a metronidazole gel.

A six-month study found that after rosacea was brought under control with oral antibiotics and metronidazole, using metronidazole gel alone maintained control of symptoms for a significant number of patients.

You should probably avoid alcohol while taking oral metronidazole because an antabuse-like reaction has been reported. Antabuse is a drug used in treating alcoholics. Drinking alcohol while on antabuse can make you very sick—apparently so can alcohol on metronidazole.

You may want to discuss other possible side effects with your dermatologist if metronidazole is prescribed over a long term. It should probably be avoided during pregnancy.

TRETINOIN

This antibiotic is sometimes prescribed for severe cases of rosacea or cases that resist other therapies. It does more than fight bacteria. It increases blood flow to the skin because new blood vessels are formed. It also increases the production of dermal collagen. Tretinoin reduces the production of melanin and distributes it more evenly throughout the skin. It can make the skin red, dry and sensitive to sunlight.

Once source reported that isotretinoin can cause birth defects, so women who take it must be on birth control pills during treatment. In fact, the recommendation was that you start birth control pills a month before taking isotretinoin, continue with the birth control pills all during treatment, and take them for at least two months after you stop taking isotretinoin. Talk to your doctor about this if tretinoin is prescribed.

OTHER DRUGS USED FOR ROSACEA

While antibiotics have been prescribed for a long time, dermatologists are studying other drugs for treating rosacea. Here are some that have demonstrated positive effects. If you are particularly concerned about long-term antibiotic use, discuss these drugs with your doctor.

RETINALDEHYDE

This relative of retinoic acid was found to alleviate rosacea erythema and telangiectasia without irritating the skin. Retinoic acid had previously been found beneficial in treating the vascular aspects of rosacea, but it aggravated erythema, skin dryness, burning and stinging.

A formula of 0.05% retinaldehyde reduced erythema in 70% of patients after six months of treatment in a study performed in France. The effect on telangiectasia was less clear-cut. At five months, 62% showed improvement; but at six months only 46% did. Because the study was conducted during winter through summer months, weather-related factors may have affected the results.

There are various theories as to what retinaldehyde does to relieve rosacea symptoms. One is that topical retinaldehyde benefits photo-damaged skin, so it may be good for the skin's underlying tissues. Retinaldehyde may help expel the *Demodex* mite that has been involved with rosacea.

Yet another theory is that the redness may be masked by the epidermis thickening that occurs with retinaldehyde use. There is also speculation that retinaldehyde has a direct effect on capillaries, but more research is needed before the connection between the effect on the capillaries and rosacea symptoms is clear.

CORTICOSTEROIDS

Topical corticosteroids are effective treatment for rosacea inflammation, but in long-term use they tend to atrophy the skin. While they may be a good idea to bring serious symptoms under control, topical corticosteroids should probably not be used as regular treatment.

Of course, there may be other reasons specific to you that make topical corticosteroids appropriate for you. If your doctor prescribes them, you could ask about possible skin atrophy and see what the response is.

AZELAIC ACID

This naturally occurring acid shows promise as a rosacea treatment. It creates fewer side effects and demonstrates less chance of bringing on allergic reactions than antibiotics do.

A Canadian study comparing azelaic acid to topical metronidazole found little difference in effectiveness treating papules and pustules. Research subjects reported significantly improved erythema appearance after 15 weeks of azelaic acid use. Most of the study participants preferred azelaic acid over metronidazole based on comfort, dryness, cosmetic appearance and greasiness.

LASER THERAPY

Pulse tunable dye laser therapy can be used to treat telangiectasia, redness, flushing and rhinophyma.

Researchers in Wales recorded dramatic results after an average of just three treatments. Patients reported reductions of 75% in telangiectasia, 55% reduction of flushing and 50% reduction in redness. Telangiectasia was reduced in as few as one or two treatments.

Laser therapy is effective in removing the build-up of extra tissue on the nose in rhinophyma, too.

You may want to discuss this option with your dermatologist.

DEALING WITH DOCTORS

While we are talking about doctors, here are some tips to make consultations with your doctor more fruitful. Many of us are intimidated by folks who managed to survive medical school and internship. Some of us get our medical care through HMOs (health maintenance organizations), which can take on the flavor of an assembly line because doctors seem to have quotas to meet. (I must admit I don't know that HMOs require quotas any more than I know for sure that highway patrol officers have traffic ticket quotas to fill, but the rumors abound.)

Few of us get to go see Marcus Welby when we need medical attention. Rather, we are more likely to meet with an over-worked, but competent physician. You need to take an active role in the doctor/patient relationship. You need to ask questions so you will have the information you need to make informed decisions about your care.

I find it helps to write down my questions on an index card before I leave the house. In the car, I usually come up with a couple more. The last time I saw my doctor, she caught me scribbling on a card when she walked into the examining room.

You need to take an active role in the doctor/patient relationship.

Here are some basic questions you may want to ask your doctor:

Will you explain in layman's terms what is happening to my body [because of my disease or condition]?

How will the treatment/medication affect my body?

What effects can I expect to see from the treatment or medication you are prescribing?

What are the possible side effects of the medication?*

Are there special instructions for taking/applying the medication?* Full or empty stomach? Morning or evening? At what point in skin care routine?

Are there any reactions to the medication I should watch for?*

How soon should I expect to see results?

What is my long-term prognosis?

If my condition/disease gets worse, what are the medication/treatment options?

What life style changes can I make to improve my health/condition?

Are there any foods or over-the-counter medicines I should avoid while on medication?*

How long should I expect to be under treatment?

Will I ever play the piano?

*I make a particular point to jot down notes about the doctor's answers to questions with asterisks. I want to make sure I have those answers when I get home. An impression or vague memory is probably enough for some of the other questions, but details for the ones with asterisks are important.

If your doctor is one of those who is halfway out the door before you realize your time is over, put your questions in order of importance to you. I've been known to follow my doctor down the hall, card in hand, still asking questions. Obviously, those are the appointments where I didn't have to take off my clothes.

CHAPTER 14
ALTERNATIVE MEDICINE

MUCH OF WHAT WE CALL alternative medicine today used to be mainstream medicine. So-called conventional medicine is a fairly new invention in human history. It has made tremendous strides in the past 150 years and has resulted in wonderful diagnostic and treatment plans. Drugs and surgery have saved millions of lives. Most of us know someone who would certainly not be alive today without the intervention of modern medical science.

While alternative medical practitioners acknowledge the effectiveness of what they call allopathic (symptom-countering) medicine for acute diseases and trauma, they believe they are better qualified to deal with chronic conditions. Medical doctors are becoming more receptive to the holistic (whole person) approach to healing as they observe the benefits of incorporating alternative methods.

Indeed, everyone seems to agree that the best possible care comes from using both conventional and alternative (or complementary) methods. As patients take more control of their treatments, they have the opportunity to use what works for them—no matter which field it comes from.

Rosacea just may be a condition custom-made for a combination of medical science and alternative medical treatment. It is a chronic problem with no known cause or cure. Because medical science doesn't know yet just what causes rosacea, there are bound to be many theories. And plenty of treatments based on those theories. Some may turn out to be bunk, and others will be praised as being ahead of their time once research unlocks rosacea's secrets.

The alternative medicine approaches mentioned in this book are:

    acupressure

    reflexology

    naturopathy

Each section will tell you a little bit about the therapy, the theory behind it and how to apply it for rosacea relief.

I believe the alternative therapies should only be used in addition to, not instead of, treatment prescribed by a dermatologist. It is probably a good idea to check with the dermatologist to make sure none of these therapies will make your condition worse. Only you and your doctor know exactly what shape your body is in.

ACUPRESSURE

This treatment method is routinely used in traditional Chinese medicine. Traditional Chinese medicine has been practiced in Asia for thousands of years and is gaining popularity in the West.

Acupressure is a non-invasive, drug-free therapy. For that reason alone, it is worth a try.

You can learn to practice acupressure on yourself or go see a professional. This book will only offer the most basic information about acupressure. If you want to learn more, there are many good books on the subject.

THEORY OF ACUPRESSURE

Traditional Chinese medicine teaches there are 14 body pathways—called meridians—through which the body's life energy flows. Twelve of the 14 meridians are bilateral, or identically run down both sides of the body. The other two meridians run down the middle of the body. One goes down the front; the other, down the back.

There are pressure points along the meridians. Pressing these points is supposed to alter the vital force or energy called chi (pronounced *chee*).

Altering the chi can mean strengthening it, calming it or clearing a blockage of it. Specific points along the meridians effect different parts of the body. Because traditional Chinese medicine explains disease as energy imbalances in the body, the pressure points used to treat a disease may not be obvious or seem logical to us westerners. For instance, two pressure points that effect the skin are along the Large Intestine meridian.

NOTE FOR SKEPTICS

This can sound strange to people unfamiliar with traditional Chinese medicine, but some studies have found acupressure can be effective for many health problems.

Even the most skeptical have to admit to the possibility of relief from what is called the placebo effect. According to Webster, the placebo effect is "improvement in the condition of a sick person that occurs in response to treatment but cannot be considered due to the specific treatment used."

Sometimes just thinking you are doing something that will help does help

---

Conventional medicine has recognized the placebo effect for many years. Sometimes just thinking you are doing something that will help does help.

Whether you are a firm believer in traditional Chinese medicine or are looking for another tool in treating rosacea, acupressure might be worth trying.

ACUPRESSURE TECHNIQUES

Generally, you apply firm pressure to the appropriate pressure points (each pressure point is actually two points—one on each side of the body) with your thumb or finger for a minute. If you are working on more than one point, you do all the points on one side of the body before working on the other side.

Acupressure has few risks if you follow a few precautions:

never apply pressure to open wounds

never apply pressure to varicose veins

never apply pressure to tumors

never apply pressure to inflamed or infected skin

never apply pressure to areas of recent surgery

never apply pressure to areas with possible broken bones

Pregnant women should avoid applying pressure to any points in the abdominal area.

Acupressure targets the part of the body that is the root of the problem. Since no one knows what causes rosacea, it is difficult to come up with suggestions for self-help. If the idea of acupressure appeals to you, your best bet is to consult with a professional. Share what you know about what triggers your rosacea flare-ups, and together you may be able to come up with an approach.

Here are a few techniques that could help.

To help ease skin inflammation, emotional stress and hormonal imbalances, apply pressure to the point at the outer end of the elbow crease. Press firmly for a minute, then do the other elbow.

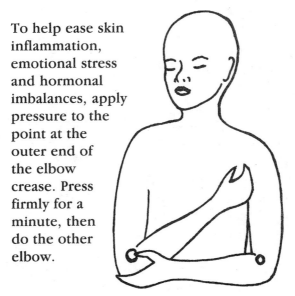

To help ease skin irritation, apply pressure between the thumb and index finger pressing against the side of the finger knuckle. Press firmly for a minute, then do the other hand.

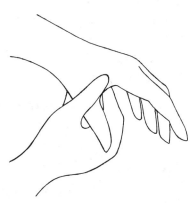

To help ease frustration, apply pressure on the highest point of the shoulder muscle halfway between the tip of the shoulder and the spine. Press firmly for a minute, then do the other shoulder.

[Pregnant women should not do this.]

To help ease emotional tension, apply pressure on the outer part of the upper chest, four finger-widths up from the armpit crease and one finger-width inward. Press firmly for a minute, then do the other side of the chest.

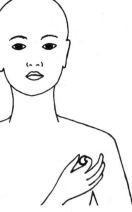

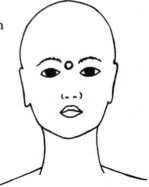

To help ease hay fever, eyestrain and indigestion [this might address histamines and ocular rosacea—who knows], apply pressure directly between the eyebrows where the bridge of the nose meets the forehead. Press firmly for a minute.

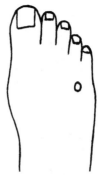

To help ease facial swelling, apply pressure on the top of the foot, an inch above the webbing between the fourth and fifth toes, in the groove between the bones. Press firmly for a minute, then do the other foot.

REFLEXOLOGY

Reflexology may be new to you, but it has been around for a long time. There is a pictograph in an ancient Egyptian physician's tomb of a man rubbing another man's foot. Reflexologists say this is the earliest evidence of the practice.

Like acupressure, reflexology uses the body's meridians as guidelines for treatment. Reflexologists picture the body with 10 meridians, instead of 14. Instead of applying pressure to different parts of the body, reflexology calls for working on pressure points that all exist in the feet and hands.

The theory is the meridians pass through the body and end up in reflex points on the feet and hands, and you can treat the entire meridian there.

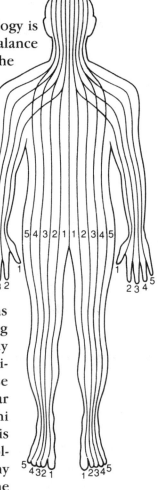

The goal of reflexology is to achieve "a state of balance and harmony." When the body is in harmony, it can heal itself. Stress is one of the biggest culprits in un-balance and dis-harmony. Reflexologists see stress as clogging up the system so the life energy doesn't flow properly through the body.

As in acupressure, a reflexologist views symptoms as signs there is something wrong with a part of the body that may not seem logically connected for those of us who are unfamiliar with the concept of chi (the life energy). There is no evidence that reflexology can harm you, so why not give it a try? [See the note for skeptics in the acupressure section.]

Reflexology can be used on both the hands and the feet. I've only included exercises for the hand, but there are plenty of books out there if you want to work on your feet.

REFLEXOLOGY TECHNIQUES

These exercises may read harder than they are to actually do. (That's a welcome change from whole body exercises that sound so easy before you try them.) Just follow each step, and after a few times you will feel less awkward.

The exercises are supposed be done on both hands. If you are right-handed, using your left hand will probably be difficult at first—and vice versa, if you are left hand-handed. Most people can learn how to do this. Don't expect to be smooth and graceful in your motions until you have practiced awhile.

The exercises are what I'll call a technique applied to a spot. The technique is what you do with your working hand. The spot is the part of the hand worked on.

It will help to practice the techniques at first, without worrying about whether you are doing the right thing to the right spot. Get the mechanics down, and then you can pay attention to the area you are working on.

TECHNIQUES

SINGLE FINGER GRIP

Rest the part of hand to be worked in the palm of the working hand. Fold the working hand fingers over the spot and press with your index finger.

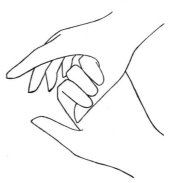

PINCH

Pinch the area to be
worked with the ends of
the thumb and index finger
of your working hand.

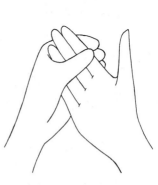

THUMBWALKING

Hold the hand to be
worked between your
extended fingers and
your thumb. Maintain
pressure with your
thumb and flex the
wrist of your working
hand. That should
increase the pressure
of the thumb.

REFLEXOLOGY SPOTS

In the exercises, you apply techniques to
places on the hand. These places are labeled as
body parts. Remember when the exercise says
to apply thumb walking to the thyroid spot, we
are talking about a place on the hand—not your
actual thyroid gland!

Some of these spots seem to have nothing
to do with the skin or the vascular system, but
they are the ones to work on. Explaining why is
beyond the scope of this book.

Here are diagrams of spots to be worked:

ADRENAL SPOT

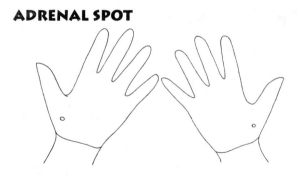

BRAIN SPOT

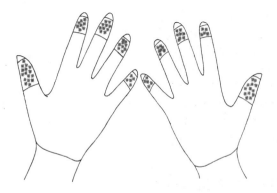

KIDNEY SPOT

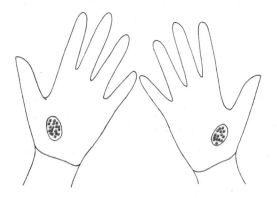

OVARY/TESTICLES SPOT

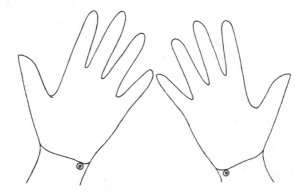

PITUITARY SPOT

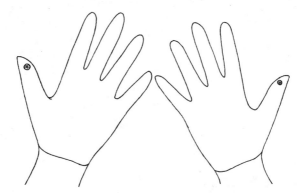

SOLAR PLEXUS SPOT

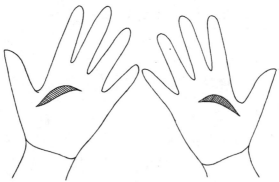

THYROID SPOT

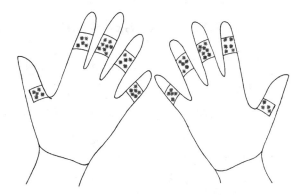

UTERUS/PROSTATE SPOT

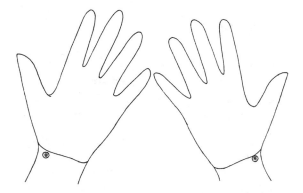

REFLEXOLOGY EXERCISES

Here are some exercises that are said to be good for the skin.

Use **THUMB WALKING** on the **THY-ROID SPOT**

Use the **PINCH** on the **UTERUS/PROS-TATE SPOT**

Use the **SINGLE FINGER GRIP** on the **BRAIN SPOT**

Use the **SINGLE FINGER GRIP** on the **ADRENAL SPOT**

Use the **PINCH** on the **SOLAR PLEXUS SPOT**

Use the **PINCH** on the **KIDNEY SPOT**

Here are some more exercises that may help the rest of the body involved with rosacea:

Use the **SINGLE FINGER GRIP** on the **PITUITARY SPOT**

Use the **SINGLE FINGER GRIP** on the **OVARY/TESTICLES SPOT**

NATUROPATHY

Naturopathic medicine "sees disease as a manifestation of the natural causes by which the body heals itself, and seeks to stimulate its vital healing forces."

The naturopathic emphasis is to treat the underlying causes of a disease or condition, instead of just to alleviate the symptoms. Instead of telling the patient to "take two aspirin and call me in the morning," a naturopathic physician carefully examines and questions the patient to try to determine what is causing the aches, pains or fever.

Naturopathic physicians do pre-med undergraduate degree work before enrolling in a naturopathic medical school where they receive training in hydrotherapy, massage therapy, therapeutic nutrition, herbal therapy, homeopathy, chiropractic, psychological counseling, and Oriental and Ayurvedic medicine. There are several accredited naturopathic medical schools in the country. Some states license N.D.s (doctors of naturopathy) as primary physicians.

Because naturopathic physicians look at the whole body when they devise a treatment plan, there is little self-help available for rosacea. The "natural" treatments in books written by naturopaths rely heavily on herbs to treat skin conditions, but rosacea is not like any other skin condition. It most closely resembles everyday acne, but acne is usually caused by bacteria.

The natural antibacterials a naturopath would prescribe for acne don't seem to do the same job on rosacea. Plus, too many herbs contain ingredients that tend to trigger rosacea flare-ups in many people.

Your best bet is probably to consult a naturopathic physician for a complete examination and treatment if this style of medicine appeals to you.

NATUROPATHY RECOMMENDATIONS

One doctor of naturopathy attributes rosacea to liver malfunction or a mineral deficiency. Her suggestions for treatment include eliminating sugar while reducing fats and red meat. She also recommends supplementing your diet with:

flax oil

evening primrose oil

beta-carotene

vitamin E

selenium

Applying grapefruit seed extract to the skin and taking grapefruit seed extract capsules will act as an antibiotic, according to this naturopath.

HYPOCHLORHYDRIA (REDUCED GASTRIC OUTPUT)

One theory for a possible factor in rosacea is reduced gastric acid output. An article published in 1920 in the British medical journal *Lancet* cited stomach analysis of rosacea sufferers that led to this theory. I've included this theory in alternative methods, because more recent research hasn't mentioned this as a possible cause or factor. In fact, excess gastric acid has been linked with rosacea during the past several years.

The symptoms of hypochlorhydria are:

a sense of over-fullness after eating

bloating, belching, burning and flatulence immediately after eating

chronic candida infections

chronic intestinal parasites or abnormal flora

dilated blood vessels in the cheeks and nose

indigestion, diarrhea or constipation

iron deficiency

itching around the rectum

multiple food allergies

nausea after taking supplements

undigested food in the stool

upper digestive tract gassiness

weak, peeling and cracked fingernails

The best way to determine if you have hypochlorhydria is a specialized test called the Heidelberg gastric analysis. The patient swallows an electronic capsule attached to a string. The capsule measures the pH level of the stomach. A radio signal transmits the pH measurement to a receiver. Then the capsule is pulled back up from the stomach.

If you don't have access to a professional equipped to perform the Heidelberg gastric analysis, the following procedure may help you determine if you have hypochlorhydria, and help supplement your hydrochloric acid output. Check with your doctor before trying this.

PROTOCOL FOR HYDROCHLORIC ACID SUPPLEMENTATION

Take one tablet (600 mg) of hydrochloric acid with a large meal. If it doesn't aggravate your symptoms, take two tablets during the next large meal. Take multiple pills throughout the meal, rather than all at once. If two tablets don't make your symptoms worse, take three tablets during the next large meal.

Continue increasing your dosage until your stomach feels warm or you reach seven tablets, whichever comes first. When your stomach gets warm, repeat the same dose at the next meal to make sure it was the tablets that caused the warmth. The warmth means you have taken too much hydrochloric acid, so at the next meal you should take one less tablet.

Once you have determined the largest dose of tablets that don't cause stomach warmth, take that number with all large meals. Take smaller amounts at smaller meals.

Your stomach should start regulating how much acid it produces, and stomach warmth should return. Cut back on the number of tablets until the warmth disappears again.

APPENDIX I
ROSACEA DIARY CHECKLIST

USE THIS FORM AT THE END of each day to identify your personal rosacea tripwires.

Date:

Check the weather conditions you were exposed to today:

❑ Sun ❑ Heat ❑ Cold ❑ Humidity ❑ Wind

Check the foods, beverages, and other items you ingested today:

❑ Spicy foods   List:_____

_____

❑ Alcohol   List:_____

_____

❑ Hot beverages   List:_____

_____

❑ Fruits   List:_____

_____

❑ Dairy products   List:_____

_____

❑ Vegetables   List:_____

_____

❑ Drugs   List:_____

_____

❑ Other   List:_____

_____

Check the conditions and activities you experienced today:

❑ Emotional stress Describe:_____

_____

❑ Physical exertion Describe:_____

_____

❑ Hot bath/sauna

❑ Warm room conditions

❑ Medical condition List:_____

_____

❑ Other   List:_____

_____

Check the substances you came in contact with today:

❑ Skin care products   List: _____

_____

❑ Cosmetics   List: _____

_____

❑ Soap   List: _____

_____

❑ Perfume   List: _____

_____

❑ After shave   List: _____

_____

❑ Shampoo   List: _____

_____

❑ Household products   List: _____

_____

❑ Other   List: _____

_____

What is the condition of your rosacea today?
❑ No flare-up ❑ Mild flare-up ❑ Severe flare-up

Did you comply with your medical therapy today?
❑ Yes ❑ No

My thanks to the National Rosacea Society for permission to use their Rosacea Diary Checklist. One-page, 8-1/2 x 11-inch checklists are available [free!] from:

National Rosacea Society
800 S. Northwest Highway, Suite 200
Barrington, IL 60010
847-382-8971

APPENDIX II
FOOD TABLE

H ERE IS A TABLE OF MOST of the foods mentioned in the food and nutrition chapters all in one place. With once glance you can see what possible triggers and beneficial ingredients a particular food has. I hope this is easier to deal with than flipping through pages looking for lists.

Remember that niacin is a mixed blessing. It is a vital nutrient, but may trigger rosacea flare-ups in some people.

FRUITS	TRIGGERS	BENEFITS
apples	Salicylate	
apricots	Salicylate	Vitamin A
bananas	Histamine	
berries	Salicylate	
cantaloupe		Vitamin A, Vitamin C
cherries	Salicylate	
citrus fruits	Histamine	Vitamin A, Vitamin C

FRUITS	TRIGGERS	BENEFITS
currants	Salicylate	
figs		Histamine
gooseberries	Salicylate	
grapes	Salicylate	
kiwi fruit		Vitamin C
nectarines	Salicylate	
oranges	Salicylate	
peaches	Salicylate	Vitamin E
plums	Salicylate	
prunes	Salicylate	Copper
raisins	Salicylate, Histamine	
raspberries	Salicylate	
red plums	Salicylate	
strawberries	Salicylate	Vitamin C

VEGETABLES	TRIGGERS	BENEFITS
artichokes		Riboflavin
asparagus		Vitamin A
avocados	Histamine	Vitamin E
beans	Niacin	Niacin, Vitamin A
beet greens		Riboflavin
broccoli		Vitamin C, Riboflavin
cabbage		Vitamin C
carrots		Vitamin A
collards		Omega-3 fatty acids
cucumbers	Salicylate	
eggplant	Histamine	

VEGETABLES	TRIGGERS	BENEFITS
green peppers	Salicylate	
kale		Omega-3 fatty acids
legumes		Copper
lima beans		Vitamin E
mustard greens		Omega-3 fatty acids
onions		Selenium
peas		Vitamin A, Vitamin C
peppers		Vitamin C
pickles	Salicylate	
potatoes		Vitamin C, Riboflavin
pumpkin		Vitamin A
pumpkin seeds		Omega-3 fatty acids, Zinc
soybeans		Vitamin E, Copper, Omega-3 fatty acids
spinach	Histamine	Omega-3 fatty acids, Riboflavin
squash		Vitamin A
squash seeds		Zinc
sweet potatoes		Vitamin C, Riboflavin
tofu		Riboflavin
tomatoes	Salicylate, Histamine	Vitamin C

VEGETABLES	TRIGGERS	BENEFITS
yams		Vitamin C
vegetables, green leafy		Vitamin A, C and E, Riboflavin

EGGS/DAIRY	TRIGGERS	BENEFITS
cheeses	Histamine	Vitamin A, Riboflavin
cottage cheese		Selenium
egg yolks		Vitamin A, Selenium
eggs	Niacin	Niacin, Vitamin E, Omega-3 fatty acids
milk		Riboflavin
sour cream	Histamine	
yogurt	Histamine	Vitamin A, Riboflavin, Zinc

GRAINS	TRIGGERS	BENEFITS
fortified cereals	Niacin	Niacin, Vitamin E, Riboflavin, Zinc
fortified breads	Niacin	Niacin, Vitamin E, Riboflavin, Zinc
oat bran		Vitamin E
rice bran		Vitamin E